Pediatric Traumatic Brain Injury
Proactive Intervention

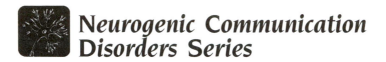

Neurogenic Communication Disorders Series

SERIES EDITOR
Leonard L. LaPointe, Ph.D.

Developmental Motor Speech Disorders
Michael A. Crary

Cognitive-Communicative Deficits Following Traumatic Brain Injury: Functional Approaches
Leila L. Hartley

Pediatric Traumatic Brain Injury: Proactive Intervention
Jean L. Blosser and Roberta DePompei

Pediatric Traumatic Brain Injury
Proactive Intervention

Jean L. Blosser, Ed.D.
Director, Speech and Hearing Center
Professor, School of Communicative Disorders
The University of Akron
Akron, Ohio

Roberta DePompei, Ph.D.
Professor, School of Communicative Disorders
The University of Akron
Akron, Ohio

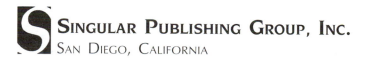
SINGULAR PUBLISHING GROUP, INC.
SAN DIEGO, CALIFORNIA

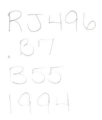

Published by Singular Publishing Group, Inc.
4284 41st Street
San Diego, California 92105-1197

© 1994 by Singular Publishing Group, Inc.

Typeset in 10.5/12.5 Goudy Oldstyle by ExecuStaff
Printed in the United States of America by McNaughton & Gunn

Library of Congress Cataloging-in-Publication Data

Blosser, Jean.
    Pediatric traumatic brain injury : proactive intervention / Jean
L. Blosser, Roberta DePompei.
        p.   cm. — (Neurogenic communication disorders series)
    Includes bibliographical references and index.
    ISBN 1-56593-168-8
    1. Brain-damaged children—Rehabilitation.   2. Communicative
disorders in children—Treatment.   I. DePompei, Roberta.
II. Title.   III. Series.
    [DNLM: 1. Brain Injuries—in infancy & childhood.   2. Brain
Injuries—rehabilitation.   WS 340 B656p 1994]
    RJ496.B7B55   1994
    617.4'81'00832—dc20   94-11315
    for Library of Congress   CIP

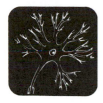

Contents

JUL 1 0 1996

DBCD - MCy 2188

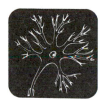

Foreword

The brain is a marvelous thing. It has been called the only human organ capable of studying itself. Although the metaphoric heart has been rhapsodized in song and sonnet much more frequently, the brain and its peculiar music has met increasing attention, not only popularly, but notably from researchers, scholars, educators, and clinicians who must deal with attempts to understand it. In fact, in the United States, the commitment to understanding the brain and its disorders has been reflected in the highest policy levels of the government, and the White House Office of Science and Technology Policy focused this attention in a report entitled "Maximizing Human Potential: Decade of the Brain 1990–2000."

When the human nervous system goes awry, the cost is enormous. Direct and indirect economic impact of brain disorders in the United States has been estimated to top $400 billion. It is impossible to measure the toll that brain disorders extract in terms of human agony from victims and their families. Each disruption of delicate neural balance can cause problems in moving, sensing, eating, thinking, and a rich array of human behaviors. Certainly not the least of these are those unique human attributes involved in communication. To speak, to understand, to write, to read, to remember, to create, to calculate, to plan, to reason—and myriad other cognitive and communicative acts are the sparks and essence of human interaction. When they are lost or impaired, isolation can result, or at the very least, quality of life can be compromised. This series is about those many conditions that arise from brain or nervous system damage that can affect these human cognitive and communicative functions. But it is not only an attempt to understand the disruption and negative effects of neurogenic disorders. As well, the authors in this series will show that there is a positive side. Rehabilitation, relearning, intervention, recovery, adjustment, acceptance, and reintegration are the rewards to be extracted from challenge. There is no shortage of these features in this series. Frustrations and barriers can be redeemed by recovery and small victories. The works in this Singular Series on Neurogenic Communication Disorders will address both the obstacles and the triumphs.

Even the Scarecrow knew. He knew the value of a brain, and he craved and sang for one. In that American film classic *Wizard of Oz*, the angular Ray Bolger chanted about neural worth (*"Dah, tah . . . daht, ta dah,tah, da daaahh . . ."*), and that is not the only lesson from the story, as you will see. The homily of hope and recovery and returning home is equally compelling. It takes no great leap of generalization to bridge these parables to pediatric head injury.

The *Wizard* metaphor and these valuable lessons are advanced in this excellent book. This publication by Jean Blosser and Roberta DePompei fills a long-recognized need. Our newspapers and local television newscasts are saturated with horrific stories of tragedy and accident. Many of these become even more numbing when we realize that children and adolescents are involved, and that families and young lives are thrown into chaos by brain damage and the inevitability of a long course of struggle and rehabilitation. Blosser and DePompei are highly regarded professionals who are experts on the cognitive, communicative, and behavioral sequelae of brain damage in young people. They cover this topic with exquisite detail and focus on the most relevant aspects of the educational challenges that are confronted during the recovery process. Along this road, which is anything but yellow-brick, these authors advance very pragmatic advice on dealing with the storms of cognition and communication that affect young people with brain injury.

This book will be helpful for all professionals who must deal with young people with brain injuries, especially those who focus on the goal of reintegration of these individuals into the community and educational system. It will be a benefit as well to both undergraduate and graduate students, to family members, and to anyone who wants to learn more about how to face the challenges intertwined with brain injury in young people. The authors have done a thorough and an empathic job in compiling this information in a readable and useful format. It has been a pleasure to have been associated with this stellar work.

Leonard L. LaPointe, Ph.D.

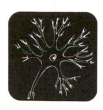

Preface

Several years ago, the two of us engaged in a lively conversation about what health care professionals "ought to know" about the school setting and what school personnel "ought to know" about the medical aspects of traumatic brain injury (TBI) to effectively meet the needs of children with TBI as they are reintegrated into the educational setting. Each of us approached the debate from our own perspective—one with years of experience in health care settings and private practice and the other with as many years working in educational settings. We each assumed the other person lacked **the** critical information needed to make sound decisions about developing goals for therapy, planning for the child's return to school, making decisions about class placement, and determining appropriate treatment and transition strategies.

As it turned out, this conversation was the beginning of a good friendship and a strong clinical team. It served as the focal point for developing our clinical interests, ideas, and philosophy about providing services for youngsters with TBI. Our thoughts have expanded beyond the walls of the school setting to include reintegration to home, work, and the community. Our understanding of TBI has increased greatly as more and more professionals and families of children with TBI have sought answers to difficult questions and requested guidance during stressful situations. We have had the opportunity to meet dedicated professionals and participate in several "think tank" experiences with national leaders in the area of traumatic brain injury. We have seen public and professional awareness of TBI increase so that youngsters with TBI are now recognized within the educational setting, and there is much concern about how to best meet their needs. The whole experience has been personally and professionally rewarding to us. It led to the invitation from Leonard LaPointe to write a book about our approach to working with children with TBI.

Pediatric Traumatic Brain Injury: Proactive Intervention is written for professionals from a variety of disciplines who are challenged daily by children and adolescents with TBI. We explain our unique, practical philosophy for planning and implementing programming for this group of youngsters. From the beginning, it was our desire to write a book that provided doable strategies for practicing clinicians. It was also our intent to promote families as integral members of intervention teams. We hope our ideas and recommendations stimulate creative problem solving, flexible programming, and interdisciplinary teaming.

The book is divided into four major parts and includes 10 chapters. Each chapter begins with an introduction and list of objectives for the reader and ends with several summary guidelines. The summary guidelines are included to alert readers to the key ideas presented. We hope practitioners will engage in dialogue with colleagues and families about these objectives and guidelines to develop a solid foundation for future programming.

Part I provides an overview of traumatic brain injury in the pediatric population and our philosophical orientation for assessment and treatment. The first chapter discusses the scope of the problem including the incidence, etiology, demographic characteristics, cognitive-communicative characteristics, and impact on the youngster's life, relationships, and experiences. Chapter 2 presents our philosophical orientation—approaching assessment and treatment from a proactive perspective. Processes for proactive planning are explained. Chapter 3 stresses the importance of working with others—family members and professional colleagues—to bring about positive changes. In Chapter 4, we discuss quality of life and transition issues and build a case for considering these factors when planning and implementing service delivery for youth with TBI.

Part II describes how to use problem-solving techniques to conduct functional assessments. Chapter 5 supports an ongoing assessment process and reviews numerous formal and informal assessment procedures. The importance of considering the influence of environmental factors on the performance of children with TBI is discussed in Chapter 6. A process for assessing environmental features is presented, including tools that can be used to conduct environmental assessments.

Part III suggests treatment approaches based on the proactive, problem-solving approach. Chapter 7 outlines general concerns to consider when planning treatment goals and selecting treatment strategies. Chapter 8 stresses ways other individuals such as family, friends, teachers, and co-workers can be directly involved in treatment. Specific, doable strategies are included. Because youngsters with TBI often experience difficulty returning to school after they are medically stable, Chapter 9 discusses problems related to school reintegration and makes recommendations for assessing the educational environment and making educational decisions.

Through a case study, Part IV illustrates a proactive approach to intervention for a child. Proactive responses to problems the child and his family experienced are provided in Chapter 10. Finally, a school reintegration planning guide is included summarizing the key points discussed throughout the book.

There are individuals we would like to acknowledge for their ideas, support and encouragement.

We thank Leonard LaPointe for his decision to include us in his series. Particular appreciation goes to Marie Linvill of Singular Publishing Group for her reinforcement and reminders as we were writing.

The text could not have been completed without the many families with children or adolescents with TBI who have shared their stories and experiences with us. Their involvement with us has shaped our family-centered approach which guides the assessment and intervention segments of the book.

Our gratitude and love is given to our families and friends, Renick, Trevor, John, Paul, Susan, and Galvin for their patience and support.

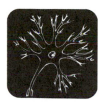

Prologue

Oh, Auntie Em, there's no place like home!
The Wizard of Oz (1939 Movie)

Dorothy's final words in the classic movie, *The Wizard of Oz*, have likely evoked strong emotional responses in all of us, as we recognize our need to be in familiar and safe surroundings. A tornado took Dorothy from her surroundings and caused her to be unconscious. Her challenge was to find a way to get back to where she had started. She traveled the Yellow Brick Road with friends who also were challenged: searching for a brain, courage, and a heart. Others, such as the Munchkins and the Wizard himself, offered advice, encouragement, and interventions. The helpers wondered if the travelers would find what they sought. The strength to meet inner challenges was found, and they came to the realization that help comes from family, friends, and strangers who can become friends. Dorothy was home.

It is instructive to see how often fiction parallels real life. Dorothy could represent any number of children who sustain a traumatic brain injury (TBI) each year. This book focuses on returning children who have sustained a traumatic brain injury to the security of their homes and communities.

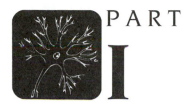
Pediatric Traumatic Brain Injury: Understanding the Problem and Developing a Philosophy of Treatment

Follow the Yellow Brick Road.
The Wizard of Oz (1939 Movie)

Meet Susan, a real-life Dorothy, as she travels the yellow brick road with her friends.

Patrolman Kenneth Fraiser was the first to arrive at the scene of the two car accident. Both cars were totaled and several individuals were injured. He was most concerned about Susan, a 16 year old who was semiconscious and sustained an injury to her head. The girls in the car were from out of state, and the officer spent considerable time in the next few hours assuring the girls and their families that the local hospital would adequately care for Susan. He worried about Susan at the time and since has wondered how else he might have helped that day.

Neurologist Thomas Struthers treated Susan in the hospital. She suffered a depressed skull fracture and cerebral contusions. An intercerebral hemorrhage was noted and surgery completed. Dr. Struthers followed Susan after surgery for about 2 months and then discharged her. He wonders if she had a complete recovery.

Family doctor John Jackson has followed Susan from reports he has received. He feels removed from her recovery process and wonders how he might have been more involved in her treatment, all of which was out of town.

Rehabilitation team members speech-language pathologist Janis Lorman, RPT Marcey Stolvey, OTR Earldean Detweiler, nurse Paul Davids, and social worker Julie Weiss met Susan in the rehabilitation facility during her 3-month stay. They did their best to stimulate all parts of her brain. They were pleased with the advances she made in all areas while she was there, but felt there were many other social and cognitive-communicative areas that were in need of remediation. They wonder how she is doing now that she is at home.

Teacher Ellie Kane has Susan in her class at the local high school. She is a little worried that Susan will not fit in with the other students because she has a head injury. Mrs. Kane has never taught a teenager with this medical problem and she isn't sure what special adaptations she might need to provide for this student. She has read the reports from the hospital and rehabilitation facility, but is uncertain about the applications of the reports to the educational setting. She thinks she and Susan will need a lot of courage to be successful this school year. She wonders if this young girl really can learn in her classroom.

Manager Dave Casanova has an employment opportunity for a teenager at the local fast food restaurant. He reads on Susan's application that she has sustained a head injury. He wonders if Susan is mentally capable of working for him and if she should be offered this after-school job. As he doesn't know much about head injury, he thinks he should pass on hiring Susan.

Parents Ken and Nora and brothers Kevin and Kerry are upset about Susan's juvenile behaviors, outbursts, poor organizational skills, inappropriate language, short attention span, and need to talk all of the time. They wonder why Susan has changed so much and when she will really be "back home."

Susan's friends, Dina, Kim, and Carrie are embarrassed by her silly talking and poor social skills. They wonder if they should continue to go to the mall with her and what the guys think of all of them these days. They wish they had more "heart" to put into maintaining a friendship with Susan.

Susan's injuries have profoundly affected all of the people who were involved with her—from patrolman Fraiser to Dina, Kim, and Carrie. They have been touched by a person who has sustained a traumatic brain injury (TBI) and they will soon learn that Susan indeed may be affected for a lifetime.

These people and Susan, like Dorothy and her friends, travel a yellow brick road of challenges. They would like Susan to "come home" and function in a world exactly as before the accident. But "getting home" isn't easy. How they will learn to accommodate to Susan's strengths and needs; what can be done to aid Susan in the classroom, at work, at home; why intervention that is functional in nature is important; and how all of these individuals might have collaborated more effectively is the focus of this book's first four chapters.

From these four chapters the reader will learn to:

1. Recognize the scope of the problem of TBI.
2. Define the incidence, causes, and physiological impact of TBI.
3. Outline the impact of TBI on a child/adolescent in home, school, work, and community.
4. Describe a philosophy for applying a proactive planning process to developing treatment for a child/ adolescent who has sustained TBI.
5. Discuss implications for collaboration and consultation that includes professionals from rehabilitation and education, family members, community members, and friends.
6. State quality of life issues and transition applications for the life cycle.

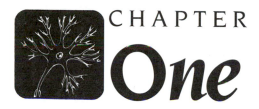

CHAPTER

One

Scope of the Problem

Interest in the child/adolescent with traumatic brain injury (TBI) has increased noticeably over the past several years. This interest seems to have been stimulated by a number of factors.

1. Injuries that would have been fatal 20 years ago are now managed by paramedics and trauma teams, with survival of severe injuries increasing annually.

2. Hospital and rehabilitation staff have recognized the need to develop programs for children/adolescents that reflect the unique needs of the population. Documentation of treatment approaches and outcomes is demonstrating how and why children improve after injury.

3. Rehabilitation and education professionals have reported that although increasing numbers of children/adolescents have returned to home, school, work, and community, treatment and supportive services of all facilities have failed to meet the demonstrated needs. Professionals' attention to descriptions of the population and their special needs has begun to provide understanding of how reintegration should occur. Education of family members, the public, and other professionals is providing a larger pool of persons knowledgeable about TBI.

4. Families and professionals have successfully advocated at national, state, and local levels for additional services for these children/adolescents because services provided were inadequate to meet the needs.

5. Laws and agency accreditation requirements now identify children/ adolescents with TBI as a disability category.
6. Prevention campaigns have increased public awareness of the possible consequences of drinking and driving; not wearing helmets when riding horses, motorcycles, and bicycles; physical abuse; reckless behavior; and risk taking.

When a child/adolescent sustains a TBI, there are immediate as well as sustained implications for the family and community throughout the life cycle. Because of enormous changes for the family, many areas of information must be understood to aid the child/adolescent develop and learn. Family and community members, peers, and rehabilitation and education professionals need to recognize and understand the scope of the problem, which encompasses:

- Terminology associated with TBI;
- Incidence and causes;
- Laws and accreditation standards specific to this population;
- Pathophysiology of the injury;
- Unique variables of TBI as they apply to children and adolescents;
- Potential impairments that can occur as a result of the injury;
- Characteristic behaviors that can contribute to difficulty in home, school, work, or community.

The remainder of this chapter focuses on developing an understanding of these issues.

Meet the Hogan Family

It is our belief that we as professionals learn much from the families with whom we work. They often provide us with insights, special information, and determination. The Hogan family consists of parents, Tom and Sharon, and children, Jason, 14; Melissa, 12; and Rachel, 10. September 6, 1992, Jason was severely injured when his bicycle was hit by a car. His mother, Sharon, has kept a journal of the family's experiences, and she has given us permission to share some of her entries with you. Her statements are scattered throughout the book in specially marked areas. She simply says. "I speak from the heart." We hope her comments provide additional insight into the truly unique world of pediatric TBI.

What Shall We Call It?
Terminology Associated With TBI

A number of terms in the literature describe injury to the brain. These terms are sometimes used synonymously, but have different meanings. Because various terms are employed, some confusion can be created. Following is a listing of terms that are often found, along with specific meanings as delineated in the law or in the literature.

Head Injury. This injury is damage to any part of the head. It is a broad term that encompasses injury from internal accidents such as stroke or external forces such as a blow to the head. Head injury can imply injuries to the face, scalp, skull, or brain (Jones & Lorman, 1989). Distinctions are made between two types of head injury: open and closed.

Open Head Injury. This is regarded as an injury in which the brain tissue is penetrated from the outside, as with an obvious wound to the head such as a gunshot wound or a crushing of the skull. The injury tends to result in localized (focal) damage and somewhat predictable impairments based on localization and degree of damage (Jennett & Teasdale, 1981; Lishman, 1973; West, Wehman, & Sherron, 1992).

Closed Head Injury. There is no open wound to the head, with damage caused by a blunt blow to the head or an acceleration/deceleration of the brain within the skull. The injury results in more diffuse brain damage with resultant variable and unpredictable consequences (Vogenthaler, 1987).

The terms "open" and "closed" also are associated with traumatic brain injury and brain injury definitions.

Traumatic Brain Injury (TBI). Several definitions for TBI are accepted. What follows is the federal Division of Special Education definition, which is in the rules and regulations for Public Law 101-476 (PL 101-476 [Individuals with Disability Education Act] {IDEA}). This definition was published on September 29, 1992 and is the guideline for state departments of education in establishing how states will provide educational services to children/adolescents. It is provided because it is applicable to children/adolescents and the services they may require in the public schools.

> "Traumatic brain injury" means an acquired injury to the brain caused by an external force, resulting in total or partial functional disability or psychosocial impairment, or both, that adversely affects a child's educational performance. The term applies to open or closed head injuries resulting in impairments in one or more areas, such as cognition; language; memory; attention; reasoning; abstract thinking; judgment; problem solving; sensory,

perceptual, and motor abilities; psychosocial behavior; physical functions; information processing; and speech. The term does not apply to brain injuries that are congenital or degenerative, or brain injuries induced by birth trauma. (Federal Register, Vol.57, no.189)

TBI generally results in diffuse axonal injury secondary to acceleration forces. This means there can be widespread damage within the cortex that can impair any variety of brain functions in unusual patterns. This damage is at the axonal or cellular level and is often not detected by brain scans. Other pathophysiologic factors that create TBI include direct laceration of neuronal tissue, edema, ischemia/hyporia, and hemorrhage.

We had to see Jason. I was not prepared for the sight I saw that night. My son was grey and looked like a corpse. We felt as if part of our soul had left our bodies. We were asked to leave . . . . and wait. Finally, the doctors came out trying to explain what had happened. Jason was in a coma with high pressure on the brain with a "closed head injury." I didn't know what a closed head injury meant until later on in the learning process. (Jason's Mom)

Acquired Brain Injury (ABI). This is a more general term that includes all types of injury to the brain, both traumatic and nontraumatic. Causes for acquired brain injury indicated by Savage (1993) include: open or closed head injury; anoxic injuries caused by reduction of oxygen to the brain from anesthetic accidents, hanging, choking, near drowning; infections such as meningitis and encephalitis; strokes; tumors; metabolic disorders such as insulin shock and liver or kidney disease; toxic encephalophy such as lead poisoning, mercury, crack cocaine, and other chemical agents.

Table 1–1 is a diagram of how Savage (1993) suggests ABI and TBI are interrelated and delineated.

Brain Damage or Injury. This is a very broad term that encompasses congenital and acquired damage to the brain. Table 1–2 outlines the broader focus of this term (Savage, 1993)

Mild TBI. This injury is synonymous with postconcussion syndrome. A very brief or no loss of consciousness is present at the time of the injury. Signs of a concussion include dizziness, headache, nausea, vomiting, lethargy, irritability, difficulty concentrating, and possible inability to recall the injury. Symptoms resolve in 90% percent of the injuries within days to several weeks. Ten percent have residuals that can last a lifetime. Implications for children/adolescents with mild TBI that does not resolve include inability to learn or organize, poor cognitive-communicative skills,

Table 1-1. Differentiation of acquired brain injury and traumatic brain injury.

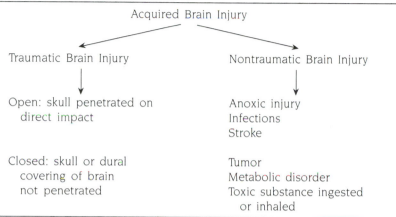

Table 1-2. Continuum of possible brain injuries.

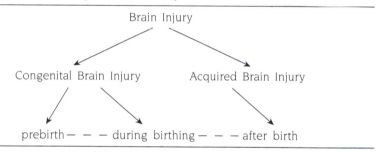

problems in maintaining concentration for school or work, psychosocial difficulties, and headaches or dizziness.

Moderate TBI. Loss of consciousness is present for up to 24 hours. Neurological signs of trauma to the brain may include skull fracture, contusions (bruises), hemorrhage (bleeding), or focal damage identified by computerized tomography (CT) or magnetic resonance imaging (MRI). Implications for children/adolescents with moderate TBI include physical weakness, cognitive-communicative impairments, difficulty learning new information, and psychosocial problems. Learning and job maintenance can be a problem for a lifetime in 33 to 50% of the population.

Severe TBI. Coma duration is longer than 24 hours. Multiple cognitive, cognitive-communicative, physical, social, emotional, and behavioral problems can exist for a lifetime for up to 80% percent of this population. Special considerations in home, school, community, and the workplace are often required.

It should be noted that the terms mild, moderate, and severe were developed to describe acute care medical conditions. These terms become less clear and less useful after the acute-care phase. About 10% of persons with mild injuries may have lifetime impairments. About 20% percent of persons with severe injuries may return to home, school, and community with minimal concerns. Therefore, no generalization about severity levels and assumptions about long-term treatment and care should be made without knowledge of individual circumstances and impairment levels. To date, research on children/adolescents has not confirmed a linear relationship between severity of injury and impact on lifetime of care injuries. However, it is implied from the National Institute on Disability and Rehabilitation Research Pediatric Trauma Registry data (1993) that the more severe the injury, the better chance that lifetime of care issues must be considered.

Who Are They? Incidence and Causes of TBI

Incidence

Each year approximately 1 to 2 million children and adolescents sustain central nervous system (CNS) injuries as a result of falls, motor vehicle accidents, sports injuries, assaults, or abuse. It is difficult to ascertain accurate statistics on the number of children and adolescents who sustain TBI, because there have been few systematic or universal guidelines developed by trauma centers, rehabilitation facilities, or school systems that provide uniform methods of record keeping. Therefore, counts differ because definitions of trauma may vary, methods of reporting are inconsistent, and facilities emphasize different aspects (medical, educational, impact on family, finances, lifetime of care issues) when obtaining data.

However, various studies have reported some statistics about children/adolescents with TBI that can be taken as indicators. One of the earliest reports from the National Center for Health Statistics (1982) stated that TBI is the leading cause of death and disability in children between the ages of 1 to 14. Kraus, Fife, Cox, Ramstein, and Conroy (1986) report that the majority of injuries are mild (about 85%) with many children not experiencing loss of consciousness.

Of the estimated 1 million injured annually, approximately 200,000 may require post-injury hospitalization and about 18,000–20,000 will be categorized as suffering a moderate to severe injury (Kalsbeek, McLauren, Harris, & Miller, 1980; Savage, 1991; Waaland & Kreutzer, 1988). Bruce (1990) stated there are about 200,000 (3–4%) of an estimated 2 to 5 million children injured annually who are hospitalized following head trauma. He reported approximately 5,000 deaths per year and estimated the mortality rate from head trauma as high as 10 per 100,000 children per year.

The National Institute on Disability and Rehabilitation Research funded program at the Research and Training Center, Tufts University School of Medicine, has compiled some of the most consistent data regarding childhood trauma. Their National Pediatric Trauma Registry compiles data from 61 medical facilities across the country. The most recent report (1993) provides information about a total of 24,573 children/adolescents covering the years 1987–1993. The data include diagnosis categories of head injury, fracture, open wound, spine, and others. Therefore, data include more than TBI. However, head injury was found to be the most frequent diagnosis (28%) following childhood trauma. Males (66%) were injured twice as often as females (33%). Age ranges were:

<1 year: 4.6%
1–4 years: 25.4%
5–9 years: 29.0%
10–14 years: 24.3%
15+ years: 16.8%

Causes of injury included motor vehicle accidents (MVA), all terrain vehicle accidents (ATV), abuse, assaults, motorcycle accidents, pedestrian accidents, stabbings, bicycle accidents, and others. The report indicates that more than 95% of children hospitalized were discharged to home or foster care. However, 37% of these children returned home with one to three impairments and 4% had four or more impairments. Impairment categories reported include vision, hearing, speech, feeding, bathing, dressing, walking, cognition, and behaviors.

These data, although reflective of all childhood trauma, indicate certain trends about traumatic brain injury consistent with other reports. Specifically, motor vehicle accidents and falls combine for approximately 80% of injuries in children; abuse data are increasing each year as a contributing factor to TBI; males are injured 2–3 times as often as females; children in different age ranges have different types of injuries (falls for preschoolers, MVA and sports injuries for teens).

As reporting becomes more accessible and the same information is accumulated across agencies, more descriptive data may be available. However, the data accumulated to date indicate that TBI is significant enough to warrant broad societal concern.

Causes

The major causes of injury to children/adolescents vary according to age, severity of injury, geographic location, and various sources of data. Bruce (1990) reports the major cause of injury to children is falls, with the major cause of death attributed to MVA. Causes of injury according to ages (Bruce, 1990; Mira, Tyler, & Tucker 1988) include:

- Infants: mishandling by caregivers: accidental dropping, rolling from changing tables, physical abuse
- Toddlers: falls, MVA, physical abuse
- Preschoolers: falls, MVA, physical abuse
- Elementary School Children: MVA, bicycle accidents, falls, injuries during play
- Adolescents: MVA (including alcohol or drug misuse), sports injuries, assault, risk-taking behaviors

The literature supports the concept that there is a disproportionate number of children/adolescents with preinjury behaviors that are factors in evaluation and treatment. These preinjury behaviors include a high percentage of teenagers who are considered risk takers and who possibly come from families where risk taking is encouraged and accepted. Additionally, Blosser and DePompei (1991), Telzrow (1991), Tyler (1990), and Ylvisaker (1985, 1993) report high rates of learning disabilities and behavior problems in children that were substantiated prior to injury. It is difficult to speculate about the reasons for such information as determination of possible TBI before school entry is not included in data accumulated about these children.

What Do the Rules Say?
Federal Legislation and Accreditation

Four recent initiatives have provided impetus for developing procedures for treatment and community access for children/adolescents with TBI. These are the Americans with Disabilities Act (ADA), PL 101-476, the Commission on Accreditation of Rehabilitation Facilities' (CARF) new standards for TBI, and expanded definitions of mental retardation/developmental disabilities (MR/DD).

Americans with Disabilities Act (ADA)

The ADA was signed into law July 26, 1990. It provides that individuals with disabilities have access to and be accommodated in employment, transportation, government activities, and communication. As TBI is a recognized disability category, children/adolescents with TBI have access to all provisions of ADA and provision of services and access should be enhanced by this law. Additional information about the law can be obtained from the U.S. Department of Justice, Civil Rights Division, P.O. Box 66118, Washington, DC 20035-6118

Public Law 101-476

In January 1991, the Education for All Handicapped Children Act (PL 94-142) was amended, renamed, and reauthorized by the United States Congress. The new act is referred to as the Individuals with Disabilities Education Act (IDEA). The reauthorized law includes a special category for youth with TBI. This law means that children and adolescents with TBI, if they qualify for special education, must be provided with appropriate education, regardless of the severity of their disability. The law also provides for transition planning to work, community, and independent living settings after graduation. This planning can begin as early as age 14. At the present time, state departments of education are developing rules and regulations for provision of service to this population. For further information about how a particular state will handle this requirement, one can contact individual state departments of special education.

The Commission for Accreditation of Rehabilitation Facilities (CARF) Standards

The Commission for Accreditation of Rehabilitation Facilities revised its requirements for individuals with TBI in organizations they accredit. The new standards became effective July 1, 1992. For the first time, CARF standards are outlined for organizations with a designated pediatric program providing services to children or adolescents with brain injury. Standards define staff composition and education, provisions for children and adolescents, provisions for family, and coordination of services for school reintegration. Following is an explanation of each of these standards.

Staff Composition and Education
a. Professionals should show evidence of orientation, preservice, and inservice training that addresses needs of siblings and peers, normal childhood development, parenting issues, and skills in working with families. These topics are listed in addition to the suggestions of education topics for professionals who treat all persons with TBI.

b. Programs must provide or make formal arrangements for services of an education specialist. Additionally, services of a pediatrician, if the child is age 12 or under, is required.

c. Core teams in a pediatric program should include a developmental specialist and a special education liaison.

Provisions for the Child/Adolescent

a. Programs should provide space, equipment, furniture, and materials according to age and developmental needs of children/adolescents.

b. Separate areas for beds should be provided for children/adolescents according to age and developmental needs and away from adults.

c. Private areas equipped with age-appropriate materials and furniture should be provided for peer and family visitation.

d. Assessment must be age and developmentally appropriate.

e. Periodic reassessment to monitor cognitive processes until the child/adolescent reaches adulthood should be completed.

f. Consumer satisfaction surveys should be adapted to elicit responses from children.

Provisions for Family

a. The family is recognized as the focal point and is to be included in all phases of planning.

b. Services, as needed, that are to be provided for the family include advocacy training, counseling, education, parent-to-parent interactions, and sibling and peer support.

Coordination of Services for School Reintegration

a. Programs should request pre-onset school records.

b. Programs should demonstrate familiarity with current federal laws specific to the education of children.

c. The program should have procedures for cooperative education and training of school and rehabilitation personnel about each other's programs, family training in educational issues and procedures, integrated planning, and involvement in the Individualized Education Program (IEP) planning process (DePompei & Blosser, 1993, pp. 245–246).

Additional information about the standards are available in the *1992 Standards Manual for Organizations Serving People with Disabilities* (CARF, 1992).

Expanded Definitions of Mental Retardation and Developmental Disabilities (MR/DD)

Several states have undertaken initiatives to develop new definitions of MR/DD. These expanded definitions may provide additional service opportunities for some youth with TBI. For example, in the state of Ohio, the definition of MR/DD now includes functional definitions of developmental disabilities. This definition states that individuals who were injured prior to age 22 may be eligible for services (such as therapies and group housing) under MR/DD boards if the persons have two or more handicapping conditions that interfere with normal life functioning. Although many children/adolescents with TBI will not qualify for services, professionals should be aware of the possibilities for providing such services and be prepared to recommend alternative options.

Also, the courts are beginning to rule on cases regarding the laws about TBI and children whose rights may have been violated. The Supreme Court of the United States in November, 1993, heard a case to determine if the parents of a child with a learning disability (as a result of TBI) are entitled to state reimbursement under the IDEA when they placed their child in a private school to obtain an appropriate education for her. The National Head Injury Foundation filed an Amicus Curiae in support of the parents. On November 9, 1993, the Supreme Court of the United States ruled in favor of the family. This case held that if parents of a child with a disability and the school board cannot agree upon an Individualized Education Program (IEP), then the parents have the option of placing their child in a private school even though the private school is not approved by the public education authorities. The parents can then seek reimbursement for tuition and related expenses, including room and board. This case does not create a right or entitlement. It only creates an option and is not without risk. If parents choose this course of action, they can only obtain reimbursement if the final court of review finds the proposed IEP was not appropriate, that the private placement was proper, and that the expense was reasonable (Denmead & Bonarrigo, 1994).

What Happened? Pathophysiological Aspects of TBI

The pathophysiological impact of TBI has been discussed by Beukelman and Yorkston (1991), Miller, Pentland, and Berrol (1990), Pang (1985), Rosenthal, Griffeth, Bond, and Miller (1990). The reader is referred to these authors for specific and detailed information.

When TBI occurs, there is the potential for considerable damage, some temporary and some permanent. The differences in the type of injury, the areas of the brain affected, and the diffuse versus focal nature of the injury accounts for the vast variability in preserved abilities in some individuals and new challenges as a result of acquired disabilities in others. What follows is a summary of the primary and secondary types of injuries that can occur and the recovery scales used to describe the resultant behaviors.

Primary Injury Mechanisms: Damage at the Time of Injury

The brain is surrounded by cerebrospinal fluid and encased in a bony skull, which provides protection (Figure 1–1). When a traumatic brain injury occurs (blow to the head, shaken violently), the force of the acceleration/deceleration moves the brain rapidly within the skull. This movement can result in several types of damage:

1. Coup-contrecoup. As can be seen in Figure 1–2 damage can be localized (or focal) to the area at the point of impact (coup). A second focal injury (contrecoup) can occur as the brain bounces from the point of impact to the opposite side of the skull.

2. Focal contusions. Portions of the prefrontal lobes and anterior and posterior temporal lobes are in close proximity to the bony prominences of the skull. When the brain is accelerated rapidly enough, it can be pushed into these bony protuberances. Bruising and an increase of blood or fluid can be seen. Brooke, Uomoto, McLean and Fraser (1991) suggest a continuum of injury, moving from accumulation of fluid only (mildest injury) to hemorrhage and formulation of blood clots (most severe injury).

3. Diffuse axonal shearing. Damage also can be widespread (diffuse). Because of the nature of the brain floating in cerebral spinal fluid, it

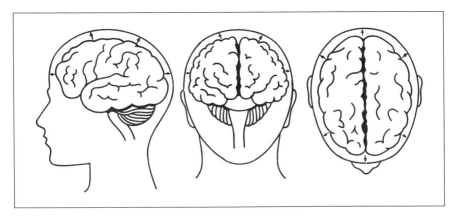

Figure 1–1. Normal brain position within the skull as viewed from the side, front, and top. *Source:* From Jones, Cynthia and Lorman, Janis (Revised Edition–1994). *Traumatic Brain Injury: A Guide for the Patient and Family.* Stow, OH: Interactive Therapeutics Inc. Reprinted with permission.

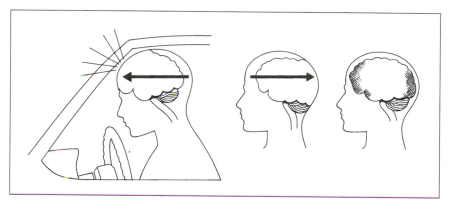

Figure 1–2. Multiple injuries to the brain. Injury occurring at the point of impact and opposite of point as the brain bounces within the skull. *Source*: From Jones, Cynthia and Lorman, Janis (Revised Edition–1994). *Traumatic Brain Injury: A Guide for the Patient and Family*. Stowe, OH: Interactive Therapeutics Inc. Reprinted with permission.

moves slightly slower than the skull. Since the brain sits on the spinal cord, much like a flower on its stem, twisting or swirling movements can produce a forcing together of tissues, a pulling apart of tissues and a tearing or shearing of axonal fibers (Figure 1–3).

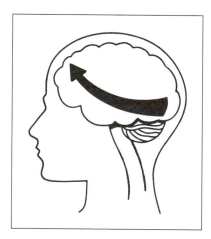

Figure 1–3. Rotational injury to nerve fibers in the brain result as the brain is twisted within the skull. *Source*: From Jones, Cynthia and Lorman, Janis (Revised Edition–1994). *Traumatic Brain Injury: A Guide for the Patient and Family*. Stow, OH: Interactive Therapeutics Inc. Reprinted with permission.

Axonal damage occurs at the cellular level and may not be seen on CT or MRI scans. However, when the brain is examined microscopically, small hemorrhages or lesions with reaction bulb formations of axons are seen. Additionally, microglial clusters also are present, which indicate damage has occurred. Axons are critical to transmission of information in the brain, as well as maintenance of consciousness. Diffuse axonal injury (DAI) often results in coma. DAI is also a major contributor to the overall cognitive damage that can occur. Ylvisaker (1993) indicates outcomes from diffuse axonal damage can include slowdown in processing of information, difficulty alerting, attention problems, slowed and more labored gait or speech, fatigue, and difficulty integrating information and organizing responses. This type of damage also forms the basis for understanding the uniqueness of the injury from one person to another, as no two persons will suffer identical diffuse damage.

Secondary Mechanisms of Injury: Complications After Initial Injury

1. Edema. Swelling occurs at the time of injury and can continue for some time afterward. In closed-head injuries, there is no room for swelling tissue to expand beyond the cranial vault, resulting in an increase in intracranial pressure that can contribute to a decline in consciousness. Treatment usually includes medication to reduce swelling and, occasionally, surgery to remove a portion of the skull or brain to alleviate the pressure of the swelling brain against the skull.

2. Hypoxia. Abnormally low amounts of oxygen are supplied to the brain. This is particularly of concern to areas of the brain such as the hippocampus (memory), basil ganglia (movement), and end arterial supply areas of the cerebral cortex and cerebellum (feeding of the cortex).

3. Hemorrhage or hematoma. As a result of the contusion or bruising process, bleeding or development of blood clots continue to be a concern. Any disruption of the cerebral blood flow or its regulation can contribute to additional brain damage.

4. Seizures. Seizure activity after injury is a possible complication. Oftentimes, children/adolescents are placed on medication as a preventative measure. Much discussion has appeared in the literature about the preventive use of antiseizure medication and the effect these medications may have on an already slowed processing system (Cope, 1987). Additional research is needed to determine what the best course of action might be.

Recovery Scales

The literature abounds with attention to measures of recovery from coma and descriptive information about recovery from coma. These scales are widely used clinically and are a frequent part of research reports. The three most commonly used scales are the Glasgow Coma Scale (GCS),(Jennett & Teasdale, 1981); the Ranchos Los Amigos Scale of Cognitive Functioning (Hagen & Malkmus, 1979); and the duration of posttraumatic amnesia (PTA) as evaluated by the Children's Orientation and Amnesia Test (COAT) (Ewing-Cobbs et. al., 1984).

I had to keep thinking of ways to help Jason, to stay one step ahead. I contacted his friends and asked them to tape conversations for him. I called his favorite radio station and asked the DJ to dedicate a song to him. I played the dedication and tapes to him while he was still in a coma. Those familiar voices helped my son to remember who he was. (Jason's Mom)

Glasgow Coma Scale

This scale is employed in acute care facilities. It is used to determine level of consciousness and is a tool for localizing neurologic findings. Table 1–3 is a description of the scale.

Ranchos Los Amigo Scale of Cognitive Functioning

This scale is a multivariate description of behaviors as a person emerges from coma (Hagen & Malkmus, 1979). It offers general behaviors that can be anticipated during each stage. It should be noted that a person

Table 1–3. Glascow Coma Scale.

Eye Opening		
spontaneous	E	4
to speech		3
to pain		2
nil		1
Best motor response		
obeys	M	6
localizes		5
withdraws		4
abnormal flexion		3
extensor response		2
nil		1
Verbal response		
orientated	V	5
confused conversation		4
inappropriate words		3
incomprehensible sounds		2
nil		1

Coma score (E + M + V) = 3 to 15

Source: From Jennett, B., & Teasdale, G. (1981). *Management of head injuries*, p. 78. Philadelphia: F. A. Davis Company. Reprinted with permission.

can be in more than one stage at a time. It is also possible to plateau in a stage and remain for long periods of time or to move rapidly through all stages. Malkmus (1982) added cognitive-communicative descriptions for each level of recovery. Table 1–4 is a summary of this combined scale.

These scales are primarily for individuals 14 years and older. The Rancho staff has adapted a scale for children under 14 years of age. This scale is not as widely used or accepted as those for older patients. Many professionals believe that children's developmental differences complicate accurate interpretation of the scale for the very young.

Posttraumatic Amnesia (PTA)

PTA is defined as the time from coma until the individual is oriented to time, place, and person. The Children's Orientation and Amnesia Test (COAT) is often employed to evaluate PTA in children. The full test is available in Rosen and Gerring (1986, pp. 129–130).

Concerns about use of PTA as a long-term measure are expressed by some professionals, because a child can be oriented to person, time, and place, but remain unable to use this information functionally in home, school, or community.

What Is It Like? Characteristics of TBI

In pediatric TBI, a variety of physical, social, behavioral, cognitive, communicative, and emotional problems are apparent. Various authors (Begali, 1987; Blosser & DePompei, 1992; Cohen, 1986, 1991; DePompei & Blosser, 1987, 1991a, 1991b, 1993; Gerring & Carney, 1992; Lehr & Savage, 1990; Savage, 1991; Telzrow, 1987; Tyler, 1990; Ylvisaker, 1985, 1993; Ylvisaker, et al., 1990; Ylvisaker & Sezekeres, 1994) outline characteristic behaviors observed in children or adolescents with TBI. Table 1–5 is a compilation of the behaviors and impairment areas reported for youth with TBI (DePompei & Blosser, 1993).

Certain processes are important for communication. These include:

- **Attention:** The ability to maintain awareness long enough to respond to a stimulus. Often children/adolescents have poor vigilance and are unable to sustain attention long enough to respond. Dividing attention in the presence of two or more stimuli also is a frequent problem. Attention is critical to the assessment and intervention process and must be a primary consideration of language competencies after TBI.

- **Long-Term Memory:** The ability to mentally record and store events, feelings, actions and reactions, and then recall them as needed. Semantic (memory for facts) and episodic (memory for temporal events) memory skills may be lacking after TBI.

Table 1–4. Rancho Scale of Cognition and Language, levels of cognitive functioning and associated linguistic behaviors.

Level I. No response

General Behaviors

Patient appears to be in a deep sleep and is completely unresponsive to any stimuli presented.

Linguistic Behaviors

Receptive: No evidence of processing of linguistic input.

Expressive: Absence of verbal and gestural expression.

Level II. Generalized Response

General Behaviors

Patient reacts inconsistently and nonpurposefully to stimuli in a nonspecific manner. Responses are limited in nature and are often the same regardless of stimulus presented. Responses may be physiological changes, gross body movements and vocalization. Responses are likely to be delayed. The earlier response is to deep pain.

Level III. Localized Response

General Behaviors

Patient reacts specifically but inconsistently to stimuli. Responses are directly related to the type of stimulus presented, as in turning head toward a sound or focusing on an object presented. The patient may withdraw an extremity and vocalize when presented with a painful stimulus. He or she may follow simple commands in an inconsistent, delayed manner, such as closing eyes, squeezing or extending an extremity. Once external stimuli are removed, the patient may lie quietly. He or she may also show a vague awareness of self and body by responding to discomfort such as pulling at the nasogastric tube or catheter or resisting restraints. He or she may show a bias toward responding to some persons, especially family and friends, but not to others.

Linguistic Behaviors

As the patient progresses through this phase, linguistic behaviors emerge.

Receptive: Progresses from localizing to processing, retaining and following simple commands which elicit automatic responses; inconsistent and delayed. May demonstrate limited graphic processing.

Expressive: Emergence of automatic verbal and gestural responses. Negative head nods, requiring less head control, before positive. Single word expressions or several words used as "holophrastic" responses. Expression is dependent upon elicitation by an external stimulus.

(continues)

Table 1–4. *(continued)*

Level IV. Confused-Agitated

General Behaviors

Patient is in a heightened state of activity with severely decreased ability to process information. He or she is detached from the present and responds primarily to his or her own internal confusion. Behavior is frequently bizarre and nonpurposeful relative to the immediate environment. He or she may cry out or scream out of proportion to stimuli even after removal, may show aggressive behavior, attempt to remove restraints or tube or crawl out of bed in a purposeful manner. He or she does not discriminate among persons nor objects and is unable to cooperate directly with treatment efforts. Verbalization is frequently incoherent or inappropriate to the environment. Confabulation may be present; patient may be hostile. Gross attention to environment is very brief and selective attention often nonexistent. Being unaware for present events, patient lacks short term recall and may be reacting to past events. He or she is unable to perform self-care activities without maximum assistance. If not disabled physically, he or she may perform automatic motor activities such as sitting, reaching, and ambulating as part of the agitated state but not as a purposeful act nor on request, necessarily.

Linguistic Behaviors

Severe disruption of frontal-temporal lobes, and resultant confusion, becomes apparent.

Receptive: Marked disruption of integrity of auditory mechanism, with severe decreases in ability to maintain temporal order of phonemic events, rate of processing and ability to attend to, retain, categorize and associate information. Graphic processing is equally affected. Compounded by disinhibition and inability to inhibit response to internal stimuli.

Expressive: Marked disruption of phonological, semantic, syntactic and suprasegmental features. Characterized by disinhibition, incoherence; bizarre and unrelated to environment. Frequently, literal, verbal and neologistic paraphasias are present, with disturbance of logico-sequential features and incompleteness of expression. Prosodic features are disturbed secondary to inability to cognitively monitor and adjust rate, pitch, vocal intensity, etc.

Level V. Confused-Inappropriate

General Behaviors

Patient appears alert and is able to respond to simple commands fairly consistently. However, with increased complexity of commands or lack of any external structure, responses are nonpurposeful, random or, at best,

Linguistic Behaviors

Marked by presence of linguistic fluctuations according to degree of external structure present and familiarity-predictability of linguistic events.

fragmented toward any desired goal. He or she may show agitated behavior but not on an internal basis, as in Level IV; rather as a result of external stimuli and usually out of proportion to the stimulus. The patient has gross attention to the environment, is highly distractible and lacks ability to focus attention to a specific task without frequent redirection. With structure he or she may be able to converse on a social-automatic level for short periods of time. Verbalization is often inappropriate; confabulation may be triggered by present events. Memory is severely impaired, with confusion of past and present in reaction to ongoing activity. Patient lacks initiation of functional tasks and often shows inappropriate use of objects without external direction. He or she may be able to perform previously learned tasks when structured, but is unable to learn new information. He or she responds best to self, body, comfort and, often, family members. The patient usually can perform self-care activities with assistance and may accomplish feeding with supervision. Managment on the unit is often a problem if the patient is physically mobile as he or she may wander off, either randomly or with vague intention of "going home."

Receptive: Processing improved, with increased ability to retain temporal order of phonemic events, but persistence of semantic and syntactic confusions. Length of retained input is limited to phrases or short sentences. Rate, accuracy and quality remain significantly reduced, with auditory processing better than graphic.

Expressive: Disruption of phonological, semantic, syntactic and prosodic features persists. Characterized by disturbance of logico-sequential features; irrelevancies, incompleteness, tangential, circumlocutious and confabulatory expression. Decrease in literal paraphrasias; neologisms and/or verbal paraphasias persists. Length of utterance may be decreased or increased, depending on inhibition-disinhibition factors. Expressive responses are stimulus-bound. Word retrieval deficits become apparent, as characterized by delay, generalization, description, semantic association and/or circumlocution. Disruption of syntactic features evident beyond concrete level of expression or with increase in length of output. Graphic expression is severely limited; gestural expression is limited and incomplete.

Level VI. Confused-Appropriate

General Behaviors

Patient shows goal directed behavior, but is dependent on external input for direction. Response to discomfort is appropriate and he or she is able to tolerate unpleasant stimuli, e.g., NG tube, when need is explained. He or she follows simple directions consistently and shows carryover for

Linguistic Behaviors

Receptive: Processing remains delayed, with difficulty retaining, analyzing-synthesizing input. Processing of auditory input improves to compound sentence level; graphic stimuli processed at short sentence level. Self-monitoring capacity emerges.

(continues)

Table 1–4. *(continued)*

tasks learned; e.g., self-care. He or she is at least supervised with old learning; unable to maximally assisted for new learning with little or no carry-over. Responses may be incorrect due to memory problems but are appropriate to the situation. They may be delayed to immediate and he or she shows decreased ability to process information with little or no anticipation or prediction of events. Past memories show more depth and detail than recent memory. The patient may show beginning awareness of the situation by realizing he or she doesn't know an answer. He or she no longer wanders and is inconsistently oriented to time and place. Selective attention to tasks may be impaired, especially with difficult tasks and in unstructured settings, but is now functional for common daily activities. The patient may show vague recognition of some staff and has increased awareness of self, family and basic needs.

Expressive: Expression reflects internal confusion-disorganization, but is appropriate to situation or idea. Information retrieval and expression reflects significantly reduced new learning and displacement of temporal and situational contexts. Social automatic expression is essentially intact; expression remains stimulus-bound. Tangential, irrelevant responses are diminished in familiar, predictable situations; re-emerge in open-ended communicative situations requiring referential language. Confabulatory responses and neologisms extinguish. Literal paraphasia persists only if specific apraxia is present. Word retrieval errors occur in referential language but seldom in confrontation naming. Length of utterance remains reduced unless marked disinhibition is present, resulting in inability to channel flow of ideas-expression. Limited graphic expression emerges. Gestural expression increases. Prosodic features reflect "voice of confusion": equal stress, monopitch and monoloudness.

Level VII. Automatic-Appropriate

General Behaviors

Patient appears appropriate and oriented within hospital and home settings, goes through daily routine automatically but robot-like, with minimal to absent confusion and has shallow recall for what he or she has been doing. He or she shows increased awareness of self, body, family, food, people and interaction in the environment. The patient has superficial awareness of but lacks insight into his condition, decreased judgment and problem solving and lacks realistic planning for the future. He or she shows carryover for new learning at a decreased rate. The

Linguistic Behaviors

Majority of linguistic behaviors appear "normal" within familiar, predictable, structured environments, but persistent deficits are apparent in open-ended communication and less structured settings.

Receptive: Reductions persist in rate and quality of auditory and graphic processing regarding length, complexity and competitive stimuli. Retention improves to short paragraph level, but difficulty discerning salient features, organizing/integrating input and absence of detail persists.

patient requires at least minimal supervision for learning and safety purposes. He or she is independent in self-care activities and supervised in home and community skills for safety. With structure, he or she is able to initiate tasks or social and recreational activities in which there is now interest. His or her judgment remains impaired. Prevocational evaluation and counseling may be indicated.

Expressive: Automatic level of language is apparent in referential communication, verbal reasoning; primarily self-oriented and concrete. Tangential expression and irrelevancies evidenced in abstract linguistic attempts. Word retrieval errors persist, with reduced frequency. Length of utterance and gestural expression approximate normal. Graphic expression increases to short paragraphs; syntactic disorganization, simplistic, with irrelevancies. Prosodic features remain aberrant.

Level VIII. Purposeful-Appropriate

General Behaviors

Patient is alert and oriented, and is able to recall and integrate past and recent events and is aware of and responsive to his culture. He or she shows carryover for new learning if acceptable to him or her and his other life role and needs no supervision once activities are learned. Within his or her physical capabilities, the patient is independent in home and community skills. Vocational rehabilitation, to determine ability to return as a contributor to society, perhaps in a new capacity, is indicated. He or she may continue to show decreases relative to premorbid abilities in quality and rate of processing, abstract reasoning, tolerance for stress and judgment in emergencies or unusual circumstances. His social, emotional and intellectual capacities may continue to be at a decreased level for him, but functional within society.

Linguistic Behaviors

Language capacities may fall within normal limits. Otherwise, problems persist in competitive situations and in response to fatigue, stress and emotionality reducing effectiveness, efficiency and quality of performance.

Receptive: Rate of processing of auditory and graphic input remains reduced but unremarkable upon testing. Retention span remains limited at paragraph level, but improved with use of retrieval-organization strategies. Analysis, organization, integration are reduced in rate and quality.

Expressive: Syntactic and semantic features fall within normal limits; verbal reasoning, abstraction remain reduced. Graphic expression usually falls below premorbid level. Prosodic features fall within normal limits unless dysarthria is present.

Source: Adapted from Malkmus, 1981. Cognition and Language, Models & Techniques of Cognitive Rehabilitation, Second Annual International Symposium, Indianapolis, Indiana.

- **Short-Term, or Working Memory**: Information that is not stored, but is used to process and appreciate stimuli, allowing the ability to follow directions or hold information in memory long enough to act on it. Short-term, or working memory, is often impaired in TBI. This has an impact on the ability to follow directions in school or work and is often the type of memory problem that is the most difficult for persons with TBI.

- **Executive Functioning**: The ability to self-analyze and monitor and to set goals and determine success measures. Executive functioning develops throughout childhood. TBI can interfere with the development of self-awareness and insight and, therefore, affect executive functioning.

- **Reasoning and Problem Solving**: The use of a series of steps to arrive at a solution. TBI can interfere with the natural development of deductive, inductive, and analytic reasoning in children.

- **Anomia**: Difficulty with word retrieval or naming tasks. This can be caused by poor memory, inappropriate processing, lack of vocabulary development over time, or weak categorization and association abilities. Many children/adolescents with TBI demonstrate this characteristic.

- **Hyperverbal Speech**: Inappropriate control of the conversation by maintaining long spoken sentences containing little relevant content. Poor pragmatic skills, inability to recognize or react to others' nonverbal communication, or lack of self-monitoring skills are often present.

- **Tangential Speech**: Inability to remain on a specified topic or to return to a topic area. Poor pragmatic skills, including topic drift during conversation or narrative discourse, as well as inability to recall may be seen.

- **Confabulation**: Untrue aspects of connected speech, story telling, filling in information. This may be attributed to memory impaired for recalling actual information.

- **Expressive Speech or Language Problems**: Children may exhibit difficulty formulating phonemes, words, or sentences after a TBI. Motor impairment may be present, dysarthria or cognitive processes may be impaired, and the ability to recall and retrieve words or formulate sentences may be problematic. Effects of this difficulty can extend to the printed word and affect both reading and writing.

- **Receptive Language Problems**: Inability to follow directions, process auditory information. Central auditory processing or attentional difficulties can create receptive problems. Additionally, peripheral hearing loss may occur and always should be evaluated as a possible contributor to receptive problems.

- **Cognitive-Communicative Disorders**: The American Speech-Language-Hearing Association (ASHA, 1988) defines cognitive communicative impairments as, "Those communicative disorders that result from deficits in linguistic and non-linguistic cognitive processes" (p.79). ASHA further states that there are many cognitive processes that underlie language development. When these processes are impaired, deficits in language will be the outward manifestation reflected by the underlying problems. These cognitive processes may include:

Impaired attention, perception and/or memory;

Inflexibility, impulsivity, disorganized thinking;

Difficulty processing complex information;

Problems learning new information;

Inefficient retrieval of stored information;

Ineffective problem solving or judgment;

Inappropriate social behavior (pragmatics); and

Impaired executive functioning

Jason continues to react on impulse without thinking of any danger. He has no fears. He's like a small child. The aide has to watch him all the time. He's trying to prove to the world he can do anything. I am glad he has the spirit and wouldn't have it any other way. It's because of that spirit he has come this far. However, the timing of his spirit is off! (Jason's Mom)

Cognitive-communicative impairments are the predominant types of language disturbances related to TBI. Del Toro (1991) states that the disruption of underlying cognitive processes is related to the pattern of injury found in TBI. Ylvisaker and Szekeres (1986) report that widespread diffuse shearing lesions in the cortex are associated with disorders of attention, concentration, and efficient information processing, indicating the neurological basis underlying the cognitive-communicative impairments.

The impairments in cognitive-communicative abilities of children/adolescents with TBI are manifested in ineffective learning and performance in home, school, work, or community and poor social interaction. These poor performances in communication may be responsible for the reports of unsuccessful reintegration into the community and may ultimately interfere with acceptance by family and peers.

All of the characteristics listed in Table 1–5 can be identified in other populations of children/adolescents with disabling conditions. Many simi-

***Table* 1–5.** Types of impairments in individuals with TBI.

The following characteristics can occur in an individual with a head injury. They can occur in a number of combinations, and no two individuals will demonstrate the same patterns.

Medical:

Complications may include
—Seizures
—Bowel and bladder control
—Pain
—Orthopedic

Sensory:

Consider that there may be difficulty with
—Vision
—Smell
—Touch
—Hearing
—Taste
—Kinesthesia

Physical:

Look for impairments in
—Mobility
—Strength
—Coordination
—Endurance
—Hearing
—Balance
—Skilled motor activities

Perceptual-motor:

Think about involvement in
—Visual neglect
—Visual field cuts
—Motor apraxia
—Motor speed
—Motor sequencing

Cognitive-communication:

Observe for problems with
—Articulation
—Tangential speech
—Hyperverbal speech
—Confabulations
—Anomia (word finding)
—Language
—Abstraction
—Reading comprehension
—Writing

Cognitive:

Watch for difficulty in
—Memory (both short- and long-term)
—Thought processes
—Conceptual skills
—Problem solving
—Attention
—Concentration
—Self-awareness of abilities
—Egocentric thinking
—Inability to anticipate and plan for the future
—Inability to plan action to meet desired goals
—Self-regulation difficulties

Behavior:

Be aware that brain injury may account for
—Impulsivity
—Poor judgment
—Disinhibition
—Dependency
—Anger outbursts
—Poor motivation
—Denial
—Depression
—Emotional lability
—Apathy
—Lethargy

Social:

Sensitize yourself to know that the survivor may
—Not learn from peers
—Not learn from social situations
—Withdraw
—Distract in noisy surroundings
—Become lost even in familiar surroundings
—Be bossy and argumentative
—Demonstrate poor responsibility and dependency
—Misperceive social actions and events
—Be easily influenced by others

Other behaviors that may be displayed include:
—Loneliness
—Restlessness
—Stubbornness
—Mood changes without reason
—Perseveration
—Unrealistic plans for the future
—Sexually inappropriate behaviors
—Hypersensitivity to noise or confusion
—Reluctance to seek assistance when needed

Source: Reprinted from DePompei, R. & Blosser, J., Professional training and development for pediatric rehabilitation. In C. Durgin, N. Schmidt, & J. Fryer, Eds., *Staff development and clinical intervention in brain injury rehabilitation*, p. 234, with permission of Aspen Publishers, Inc. Copyright 1993.

larities exist in the characteristics of this population and other disabilities in children. It is on the basis of these commonalities that Ylvisaker (1993) suggested that children/adolescents with TBI should not be considered a separate disability category. He contends: (a) TBI looks like an etiology category, rather than a disability category: there are no challenges common to all members of the category—any combination of functions can be spared or impaired; (b) there is overlap in characteristics between TBI and other special education categories; (c) professionals may develop specific "TBI intervention programs" and not account for the heterogeneity within this group; and (d) noncategorical definitions would deemphasize the categorization of any disability group.

These commonalities can be used as a basis of discussion for intervention with individuals who do not understand TBI, but who have extensive experience with other populations. The development of interventions for the child/adolescent with TBI can rely on certain techniques that have worked with other populations. Selecting and applying the appropriate strategies to the special needs of individuals with TBI is essential.

Although there are commonalities that must be recognized, there also exist unique differences in the population. The extremes of behavior, as well as the unusual combinations of characteristics in TBI set this population apart, according to Begali (1987), Blosser and DePompei (1991a), Lehr (1990), Lehr and Savage (1990), and Ylvisaker, Hartwig, and Stevens (1991). Table 1–6 lists some of the notable differences that can be expected.

For a child with TBI to perform successfully in home, school, community, or work, the characteristics noted above must be understood as possible contributors to impaired communication. As every TBI is unique in the constellation of behaviors and impairments that may emerge, careful attention to the characteristics typical of a particular individual being evaluated and treated is crucial. Professionals and family members need a clear understanding of all possible skill areas that can affect the functioning of a child/adolescent.

What Can Affect Performance? Developmental Issues

One of the primary issues that must be well understood in assessment and intervention with children/adolescents is that the person being treated is not a little adult. Children and adolescents, by virtue of their youth, are in periods of rapid change that affect physical, as well as intellectual (cognition, learning, and personality) development. By the time they are well into their teens, they are in the process of learning how to learn and how to interact with situations and people in their envi-

Table 1–6. Traumatic brain injury and other types of disabilities: differentiating characteristics.

The individual with traumatic brain injury is not a "peer" of other individuals with disabilities. The learning disability has been acquired. Following are some of the characteristics that make them different. Educators and health care professionals must be aware of these differences and their effect on learning in order to appropriately plan for the reintegration process.

- a previous successful experience in academic and social settings
- a premorbid self-concept of being normal
- discrepancies in ability level
- inconsistent patterns of performance
- variability and fluctuation in the recovery process resulting in unpredictable and unexpected spurts of progress
- more extreme problems with generalizing, integrating, or structuring information
- poor judgment and loss of emotional control, which makes the student appear to be emotionally disturbed at times
- cognitive deficits that are present as in other disabilities but are uneven in extent of damage and rate of recovery
- combinations of conditions resulting from the TBI that are unique and do not fall into usual categories of disabilities
- inappropriate behaviors that may be more exaggerated (more impulsive, more distractable, more emotional, more difficulty with memory, information processing, organization, and flexibility)
- learning style that requires utilization of a variety of compensatory and adaptive strategies
- some high level skills, which may be intact, making it difficult to understand why the student will have problems performing lower level tasks
- a previously learned base of information, which assists relearning rapidly

Source: Reprinted from DePompei, R., and Blosser, J. (1993). Professional training and development for pediatric rehabilitation. In *Staff development and clinical intervention in brain injury rehabilitation*, C. Durgin, N. Schmidt, J. Fryer, Eds., p. 234, with permission of Aspen Publishers, Inc. Copyright 1993.

ronment. Three factors must be considered when a child/adolescent sustains a TBI: (1) long-term effects that can be cumulative as the child/adolescent develops, (2) delayed onset of some deficits, and (3) differences in each developmental stage, from infancy through adolescence.

Long-Term Effects

The injury can and does interfere with long-term capacity to develop. Therefore, the possible cumulative impact of deficits must be considered.

For example, if we subscribe to the ideas of Piaget (Furth, 1970; Gruber & Voneche, 1977), we must recognize that the child moves through a series of cognitive stages that influence those cognitive skills expected to be present at a particular age level. A child of 6 may be expected to develop vocabulary and add factual information that will aid the learning of new information in the future. Because of the injury, vocabulary development and retention of facts may be limited, thus hampering new learning. As the child progresses through school, demands on these learning processes increase and the child may begin to falter. It may take years to recognize a deficit such as this. Professionals who assess and treat children and adolescents need to keep this possible cumulative developmental problem in mind when completing ongoing evaluations and planning interventions.

Delayed Onset of Deficits

According to Lehr and Savage (1990), "Unique to pediatric traumatic brain injury is the possibility of delayed onset of deficits. Since an injury may affect parts of the brain that are in the process of developing or not expected to be fully functioning for a long period of time after injury, it is possible for injury effects to not be apparent for even many years after onset" (p. 302). Savage (1991) points out that a child in elementary school may perform adequately during the first several years after injury. Then, when additional demands of deductive reasoning, organization, or interpretation of written material are introduced in the upper grades, the child, as an adolescent, begins having difficulty. Because so much time has passed between the injury and the onset of problems, parents and educators may not realize the connection between the earlier TBI and the lack of performance years later.

Age Variability

Little empirical research is available regarding the impact TBI may have on each developmental stage from infancy to adolescence. Lehr and Savage (1990) provide an excellent description of infancy, preschool, elementary, and teenage levels and how a TBI may affect each developmental stage. They define the physical, emotional, and cognitive development and possible impact of the TBI on each. The reader is referred to this excellent resource for additional information.

The conference explaining the results of the evaluation hit me like a lead balloon. It was the first time someone told me that it could take at least 2 years for Jason's brain to heal. The TBI was magnified by the fact that Jason was also going through adolescent development. (Jason's Mom)

Worth Remembering

Several points about children/adolescents in various stages of development should be emphasized.

1. The vast majority of children under 5 will return home after hospitalization. Even when it appears no problems have resulted from the TBI, families of young children should be encouraged to stimulate language, learning, and exploration through play so that valuable developmental time is not lost.
2. There is wide variability in normal development of preschool children. It should not be assumed that all suspected developmental delays are a result of the TBI.
3. Even though they appear to be within normal limits following injury, children/adolescents should be reevaluated annually through all developmental years, because problems can appear at later stages.
4. Intervention programs must emphasize follow-through with community agencies or school districts so that assessments can be completed over extended periods of time.
5. Parents should be alerted to the possibility that as the child develops and there are additional cognitive, social, and emotional demands, problems related to the TBI can emerge years after an injury. They should be given resources for obtaining assistance whenever they have concerns.

The combination of developmental issues and the individual characteristics of a given TBI are great challenges to the professional providing assessment, treatment, and transitioning for the child/adolescent with TBI. In addition, understanding that impairments will have an impact on the child/adolescent's performance in the home, school, community, or work is vital.

What Can Go Wrong? Impact of the Impairments on Home, School, Community Life, and Work

Every environment into which a child/adolescent reintegrates will pose demands that will challenge performance capabilities. The child/adolescent's ability to meet the challenges of various environments depends on the nature of the impairments, personality, language skills, and temperament of the individual. All behaviors will occur within a social or learning context that involves friends, teachers, family, or community members. When there is a lack of understanding about the cognitive-communication problems, every environment poses a potential for failure.

Home

Communication in the home revolves around a variety of factors, including how the family is organized operationally relative to roles, rules, and structure (DePompei & Zarski, 1989). Other authors (Williams & Kay, 1991; Zarski, Hall, & DePompei, 1987) have dealt with the multiple concerns of the family, and it is recognized that the family is a complex unit presenting a web of possible reasons for poor interactions.

However, a major factor in the success of reinvolving the child or adolescent with TBI at home will be the youngster's ability to communicate with the family and vice versa. Difficulties reported by the family may include the inability to resume home routines, the disruption of family schedules, or the ignoring of rules and traditions.

It is especially difficult for siblings to deal with the possible inappropriate social interactions of their brother or sister. They can find their sibling's behaviors embarrassing. Siblings lack of understanding about how the cognitive-communicative deficits affect behaviors can interfere with their ability to develop positive interactions. The family will often believe that a return home signals a return to "normalcy" and when problems emerge, the family can become frustrated.

Professionals should understand the communication needs of the family and focus therapy to prepare the child or adolescent to participate as well as possible within the home communication setting. The family often can provide information that will guide the selection of situations in which to practice valuable communication skills.

School

The success of reintegrating a child with TBI to school heavily depends on the youngster's ability to communicate effectively with others and perform adequately to meet classroom requirements and situations (Blosser & DePompei, 1989). Difficulties may be reflected in the student's expression and understanding of language within the context of the school setting. Problems may arise in peer-to-peer interactions and teacher-to-student communication, as well as ability to maneuver throughout a school. Organizational skills may be a major factor in inability to maintain adequate performance in the classroom. Understanding the interaction of language and cognitive-communicative disorders with classroom performance aids family and professionals in developing plans for intervention that are appropriate to the needs of a child/adolescent.

Community Life

A third consideration is community involvement in which participation with siblings, community leaders, and/or peers is important. Many young people are involved with activities such as scouts, YMCA/YWCA, gymnastics, athletics, music, art, dance, theater, or shopping in malls. Becoming involved again in these activities with friends is a crucial element in reintegration. Communication abilities in community interactions are critical to success. Inability to maintain conversations with friends, use humor or puns correctly, respond to friends' remarks, respond to adult directions and suggestions, or behave in an acceptable manner is often a major reason for loss of friends or ability to participate in group activities. It is often the inability to learn social pragmatic skills for maintaining friends and social activities that creates problems. Yet, emphasis on these pragmatic aspects of interaction is often neglected in therapy.

Work

Teenagers often are involved in part-time jobs or are preparing for transition to full-time employment after high school. Cognitive-communicative impairments may interfere with ability to maintain a job. A teenager with TBI may be unable to follow directions, generalize from situation to situation, respond with appropriate pragmatic responses to customers or co-workers. Managers may not understand the behaviors exhibited by a teenager who is post-TBI and may not provide adequate time for learning a job. They also may not provide adequate job coaching that would help the teenager to be successful on the job. Lost employment continues to be a significant problem for teenagers with TBI.

The impact of injuries following TBI on the functioning of a child/adolescent in all environments is significant. The potential exists for the injury to interfere with all aspects of development and learning over a lifetime. By understanding the problems encountered, professionals, employers, family members, and peers can provide supportive environments for the child/adolescent to develop and grow.

Summary Guidelines

1. Vast differences exist in the type and amount of injury that can result from brain injury. No two injuries will be exactly the same.

2. Nevertheless, a number of characteristic behaviors can be outlined for a youth who sustains a TBI. Although similarities to other populations of disability exist, there are differences that need to be recognized.

3. Cognitive-communication deficits are often present when TBI is experienced. These deficits may be responsible for difficulty at home, school, community, and work.

4. Information about how these impairments affect behavior and performance in many environments must be shared with all significant persons in a child/adolescent's world.

5. The courage, brains, and heart that are needed to help children with TBI can be found in two places—the family and professionals who care and understand; the child/adolescent who uses all strength and skills to be able to say "There's no place like home."

References

American Speech-Language-Hearing Association. (1988). The role of speech-language pathologists in the habilitation and rehabilitation of cognitively impaired individuals. *Asha 29*(6), 53–55.

Begali, V., (1987). *Head injury in children and adolescents: A resource and review for school and allied professionals.* Brandon, VT: Clinical Psychology Publishers.

Beukelman, D. R., & Yorkston, K. (1991). *Communication disorders following traumatic brain injury: Management of cognitive, language, and motor impairments.* Austin, TX: PRO-ED.

Blosser, J., & DePompei, R. (1991). Preparing education professionals for meeting the needs of students with traumatic brain injury. *Journal of Head Trauma Rehabilitation, 6*(1), 73–82.

Blosser, J. L., & DePompei, R. (1992). A proactive model for treating communication disorders in children and adolescents with traumatic brain injury. *Clinics in Communicative Disorders, 2*(2), 52–65.

Brooke, M., Uomoto, J., McLean, A., & Fraser, R. (1991). Rehabilitation of persons with traumatic brain injury: A continuum of care. In D. R. Beukelman, & K. Yorkston (Eds.), *Communication disorders following traumatic brain injury: Management of cognitive, language, and motor impairments.* (pp. 15–46). Austin: PRO-ED.

Bruce, D. A. (1990). Scope of the problem: Early assessment and management. In M. Rosenthal, E. Griffeth, M. Bond, & J. D. Miller (Eds.), *Rehabilitation of the adult and child with traumatic brain injury* (2nd ed.) (pp. 521–538). Philadelphia: F. A. Davis.

Cohen, S. (1986). Educational reintegration and programming for children with head injuries. *Journal of Head Trauma Rehabilitation, 1*(2), 22–29.

Cohen, S.(1991). Adapting educational programs for students with head injuries. *Journal of Head Trauma Rehabilitation, 6*(1),56–63.

Commission on Accreditation of Rehabilitation Facilities. (1992). *1992 Standards manual for organizations serving people with disabilities.* Tuscon, AZ: CARF.

Del Toro, J. F. (1991). Language impairment following traumatic brain injury: Cognitive communicative disorders. *Journal of Head Injury, 2*(3),36–41.

Denmead, C., & Bonarrigo, D. A. (1994). A bright "IDEA" for the student with TBI. In C. N. Simkins (Ed.), *Analysis: Understanding and presentation of cases involving TBI*. Washington, DC: National Head Injury Foundation.

DePompei, R., & Blosser, J. L. (1987). Strategies for helping head-injured children successfully return to school. *Language, Speech, and Hearing Services in Schools, 18*, 292–300.

DePompei, R., & Blosser, J. L. (1991a). Families of children with traumatic brain injury as advocates in school reentry. *Neurorehabilitation, 1*(2), 29–37.

DePompei, R., & Blosser, J. L. (1991b). Functional cognitive-communicative impairments in children and adolescents: Assessment and intervention. In J. Kreutzer & P. Wehman (Eds.), *Cognitive rehabilitation for persons with traumatic brain injury*. Baltimore: Paul H. Brookes Publishing Co.

DePompei, R., & Blosser, J. L. (1993). Professional training and development for pediatric rehabilitation. In C. Durgin, N. Schmidt, & J. Freyer (Eds.), *Staff development and clinical intervention in brain injury rehabilitation*. (pp. 229–253). Gaithersburg, MD: Aspen.

DePompei, R., & Zarski, J. (1989). Families, head injury, and cognitive-communicative impairments: Implications for family counseling. *Topics in Language Disorders, 9*(2), 78–89.

Ewing-Cobbs, L., Levin, H. S., Fletcher, J. M., McLaughlin, E. J., McNeeley, D. G., Ewert, J., & Francis, D. (1984, May). *Assessment of posttraumatic amnesia in head injured children*. Paper presented to the International Neuropsychological Society, Boston.

Federal Register. (1992, Sept. 29). Definition of traumatic brain injury, 57(189). Washington, DC: Federal Register.

Furth, H. (1970). *Piaget for teachers*. Englewood Cliffs, NJ: Prentice-Hall.

Gerring, J. P., & Carney, J. M. (1992). *Head trauma: Strategies for educational reintegration* (2nd ed.). San Diego: Singular Publishing Group.

Gruber, H., & Vonech, J. J. (1977). *The essential Piaget*. New York: Basic Books.

Hagen, C. (1984). Language disorders in head trauma. In A. Holland (Ed.), *Language disorders in adults* (pp. 245–281). San Diego: College-Hill Press.

Hagen, C., & Malkmus, D. (1979, November). Intervention strategies for language disorders secondary to head injury. Short course presented at annual convention of American Speech-Language-Hearing Association, Atlanta.

Jennett, B., & Teasdale, G. (1981). *Management of severe head injuries*. Philadelphia: F. A. Davis.

Jones, C., & Lorman, J. (1989). *Head injury*. Stow, OH: Interactive Therapeutics.

Kalsbeek, W., McLauren, R., Harris, B., & Miller, J. D. (1980). The national head and spinal cord injury survey: Major findings. *Journal of Neurosurgery, 1*, 53.

Kraus, J. F., Fife, D., Cox, P., Ramstein, K., & Conroy, C. (1986). Incidence, severity, and external causes of pediatric head injury. *American Journal of Diseases in Childhood, 140*, 687-693.

Lehr, E. (1990). *Psychological management of traumatic brain injuries in children and adolescents*. Rockville, MD: Aspen Publications.

Lehr, E., & Savage, R. (1990). Community and school integration from a developmental perspective. In J. S. Kreutzer & P. Wehman (Eds.), *Community integration following traumatic brain injury* (pp. 301–309). Baltimore: Paul H. Brookes Publishing.

Lishman, W. A. (1973). The psychiatric sequelae of head injury: A review. *Psychological Medicine, 3*, 304–318.

Malkmus, D. (1982, August). Levels of cognitive functioning and associated linguistic behaviors. Presented at Models and Techniques of Cognitive Rehabilitation, London, England.

Miller, J. D., Pentland, B., & Berrol, S. (1990). Early evaluation and management. In M. Rosenthal, E. Griffeth, M. Bond, & J. D. Miller (Eds.), *Rehabilitation of the adult and child with traumatic brain injury* (2nd ed.) (pp. 21–51). Philadelphia: F. A. Davis.

Milton, S., Scaglione, C., Flanagan, T., Cox, J. L., & Rudnick, D. (1991). Functional evaluation of adolescent students with traumatic brain injury. *Journal of Head Trauma Rehabilitation, 6*(2), 35-46.

Mira, M., Tyler, J., & Tucker, B. (1988). *Traumatic head injury in children*. Kansas City, KS: Children's Rehabilitation Unit, The University of Kansas Medical Center.

National Center for Health Statistics. (1982). Advance report, final monthly statistics. *Monthly Vital Statistics Report, 31,*(6). Suppl. DHHS Publication No. PHS 82-1120. Hyattsville, MD: U.S. Public Health Service.

National Institute on Disability and Rehabilitation Research, Pediatric Trauma Registry-Phase 2. (1993). Boston: Research and Training Center, Tufts University School Of Medicine, New England Medical Center.

Pang, D. (1985). Pathophysiologic correlates of neurobehavioral syndromes following closed head injury. In M. Ylvisaker (Ed.), *Head injury rehabilitation: Children and adolescents* (pp. 3–70). San Diego: College-Hill Press.

Rosen, C.D., & Gerring, J. P. (1986). *Head trauma: Educational reintegration*. San Diego: College-Hill Press.

Rosenthal, M., Griffeth, E., Bond, M., & Miller, J. D. (Eds.) (1990). *Rehabilitation of the adult and child with traumatic brain injury*. Philadelphia: F. A. Davis.

Savage, R. (1991). Identification, classification, and placement issues for students with traumatic brain injuries. *Journal of Head Trauma Rehabilitation, 6*(2), 1–9.

Savage, R. (1993, January 6). Defining acquired/traumatic brain injury. Testimony to the U.S. Congressional Committee on Special Education. Washington, DC: Author.

Teasdale, G., & Jennett, B. (1974). Assessment of coma and impaired consciousness. *Lancet, 2*, 81.

Telzrow, C. F. (1987). Management of academic and educational problems in head injury. *Journal of Learning Disabilities, 20*, 536–545.

Telzrow, C. (1991). The school psychologist's perspective on testing students with traumatic head injury. *Journal of Head Trauma Rehabilitation, 6*(2), 23–34.

Tyler, J. S. (1990). *Traumatic brain injury in school-aged children: A training manual for educational personnel*. Kansas City, KS: University of Kansas Medical Center, Children's Rehabilitation Unit.

Vogenthaler, D. R. (1987). Rehabilitation after closed head injury: A primer. *Journal of Rehabilitation, 53*(4), 15–21.

Waaland, P. K., & Kreutzer, J. (1988). Family response to childhood traumatic brain injury. *Journal of Head Trauma Rehabilitation, 3*(4), 51–63.

West, M., Wehman, P., & Sherron, P. (1992). Applications for youth with traumatic brain injury. In P. Wehman (Ed.), *Life beyond the classroom: Transition strategies for young people with disabilities.* Baltimore: Paul H. Brookes Publishing.

Williams, J., & Kay, T. (Eds.). (1991). *Head injury: A family matter.* Baltimore: Paul H. Brookes Publishing.

Ylvisaker, M.(1985). *Head injury rehabilitation: Children and adolescents.* San Diego: College-Hill Press.

Ylvisaker, M. (1993). *Assessment and treatment of traumatic brain injury with school age children and adults.* Buffalo, NY:EDUCOM.

Ylvisaker, M., & Sezekeres, S. (1994). Communication disorders associated with closed head injury. In R. Chapey (Ed.), *Language intervention strategies in adult aphasia* (3rd ed.)(pp. 546–568). Baltimore: Williams & Wilkins.

Ylvisaker, M., Chorazy, A., Cohen, S., Mastrill, J., Molitor, C., Nelson, J., Sezekeres, S., Valko, A., & Jaffe, K. (1990). Rehabilitative assessment following head injury in children. In M. Rosenthal, E. Griffeth, M. Bond, & J. D. Miller (Eds.), *Rehabilitation of the adult and child with traumatic brain injury* (2nd ed.)(pp. 558–584). Philadelphia: F. A. Davis.

Ylvisaker, M., Hartwig, P., & Stevens, M. (1991). School reentry following head injury: Managing the transition from hospital to school. *Journal of Head Trauma Rehabilitation, 6*(2), 10–22.

Zarski, J. J., Hall, D., & DePompei, R. (1987). Closed head injury patients: A family therapy approach to the rehabilitation process. *The American Journal of Family Therapy, 15,* 62–68.

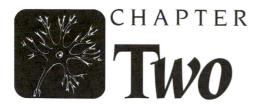

CHAPTER

Two

A Philosophy for Treatment

Because TBI results in such unique and varied impairments, many disciplines generally are involved in service delivery. Each approaches the youngster from a different perspective. Most look for deficits in the discipline's specific area of interest. This deficit-oriented approach results in service delivery that is fragmented and treatment-centered. In addition, in the school setting, it may result in inappropriate class placement and educational programming.

Current literature on treatment of individuals with disabilities argues against deficit models of intervention and in favor of treatment models that stress functional outcomes, reflect a child and family focus, and approach treatment from a unified, results-oriented front (Kreutzer & Wehman, 1991; Ylvisaker, 1993).

Intervention must be directed toward preparing youngsters to function effectively in the varied environments in which they will be living and learning—home, school, community, and work. This can be accomplished if treatment is carried out continually during interactions in real-life situations by individuals who have significant relationships with the child. Those individuals include family members, peers, school personnel, employers, co-workers, and community associates. Interactions with these types of people during formal and informal situations can offer unique opportunities for identification of needed skills and development and practice of functional behaviors.

Traditional deficit-centered clinical approaches implemented during structured or often contrived treatment sessions offer only limited opportunities for professionals to try to effect change. Such clinical strategies may not promote development of appropriate and functional skills that will help the individual meaningfully participate in activities of daily life. Rather, such strategies focus on remediation of specific impaired behaviors. Deficit-centered methods appear to be too narrow in scope and nonfunctional by design; therefore, generalization to real-life situations is limited.

A change in the service delivery model is needed to foster and achieve outcomes for students with TBI. This requires that both the process and content of treatment be targeted for change. This does not necessarily mean that new and different materials and procedures are used. Rather, the essence of this change is envisioned as a thinking and decision-making process that brings congruence to program planning.

Relatives, friends, teachers, and others all can provide important support for children and adolescents. However, contributions will be optimally effective if people are armed with doable strategies for helping. Given the opportunity to participate meaningfully in treatment efforts, others can gain confidence in their abilities to help the child succeed. Transferring the responsibility for treatment from professionals to important people in the youngster's world requires adoption of a distinctive philosophical approach that enables the professional to do so.

This chapter presents that philosophical orientation and intervention strategy. The reader will learn the key aspects of proactive planning processes and ways to apply proactive planning processes to treatment planning.

Be Forward Thinking

Rehabilitation, health care, and education professionals agree that good treatment strategies designed to achieve desired outcomes for youth with disabilities resulting from TBI are necessary and essential. Although the literature about intervention is growing rapidly, a definitive set of answers regarding the most effective methodologies and strategies has not yet been generated. As empirical evidence is lacking and research findings have not yet provided clear guidelines, we need to be creative in finding workable intervention approaches.

Sound planning and program management are necessary for any treatment program to be successful, regardless of the disability. Planning treatment programs for individuals with TBI presents service delivery teams with substantial challenges. Careful thought, organized and imaginative planning, concerted actions, and skillful management are required to achieve desired outcomes. Treatment plans also must meet expectations and requirements imposed by external sources such as funding agencies, educational agencies, and federal legislation. Responding to the diverse needs of individuals with TBI is crucial to the success of a program. Although these challenges may at times appear to be insurmountable, they also offer planners opportunities for program diversification and development.

Clinicians from a broad range of disciplines have an established history of planning treatment programs for individuals. Those plans may be labeled with various terms, but the essential components remain consistent: specification of the needs and extent of services, long-range goals and objectives, procedures for meeting goals and objectives, explanation of roles, and activities for eliciting responses and practicing new behaviors. Some of the terms used to describe the treatment plans for children are: individualized education plan (IEP), individualized family service plan (IFSP), individualized habilitation plan (IHP), and plan of care. In these designs, the plan is supposed to be tailored to meet the unique needs presented by a child in accordance with caregiver and professional recommendations. Although *the components are similar, it is the philosophy of the treatment approach that guides the content and development of a treatment program.*

In reality, the plans developed for children often focus on remediation of specific behaviors and task completion, failing to take a comprehensive, integrated view of the overall modifications needed for the child to participate as fully as possible in life's learning, work, living, and social activities. These approaches are treatment-centered and fail to see the child as connected to the world. It makes more sense to serve children by strengthening the individuals and the environments in which children interact.

In business, health care, and education organizations, leaders are adopting **quality improvement** and **strategic planning** approaches to solving problems that confront them. These approaches emphasize ongoing, interactive, analytical, innovative problem-solving methods of program management and development. The processes offer a rational, responsive perspective that also can be used for planning treatment programs. They are designed to enable key people to make meaningful decisions and contributions.

There are three key aspects of quality improvement and strategic planning that make the processes appealing as a framework for developing treatment plans to meet the needs of individuals with TBI. First, these processes are designed to enable teams of planners to **respond proactively** instead of **reactively** to problems and situations. For treatment planning, this means that problems that are likely to occur from disabilities as a result of the injury are **identified, anticipated, responded to or prevented before difficulties increase in complexity and have further impact on the youngster's performance**. Second, the processes encourage planners to **exercise creativity, flexibility, and ingenuity** in program development. This promotes **trying the untried**, freeing planners of bonds to traditional ways of thinking about and planning for treatment. Third, these planning processes stress **teamwork and involving many people in planning and implementing the program**, especially people representing diverse backgrounds and expertise. Doing this fosters **empowerment** and enables planners to **collaborate** with other persons to **access greater resources** and **provide more extensive services to a youngster**. Collaborative planning de-emphasizes competition among professionals.

To summarize, quality improvement and strategic planning processes can be used to provide a framework for the development of effective treatment programming. Following such a framework can help practitioners identify challenges that might affect success, formulate directions for change, establish priorities for treatment, define the role of important individuals, and develop strategies and plans for the successful accomplishment of goals and objectives. Following such an approach promotes the creation of an individualized treatment program unique to a student's needs and characteristics and sensitive to important environmental and people aspects. Taking a proactive stance enables planners to anticipate problems that are likely as a result of the acquired impairments and psychological changes, in addition to considering the important influence of the environments to which the child is likely to return. This framework focuses on helping professionals apply a range of treatment alternatives. It leads to programming that is relevant to a youth's individual needs; acknowledges the importance of family, peers, teachers, professionals, and community members; and facilitates reintegration.

Making It Work

To understand how to apply these proactive, quality-oriented planning processes to treatment planning, it is helpful to view the planning process as though one were planning to take a trip. Following are several questions the team needs to ask as it begins to formulate a treatment plan for the youngster with TBI:

Where is this individual now? *What is the nature and extent of the youngster's injury? From a number of perspectives, what are the resulting impairments, strengths, and needs? How do the impairments affect overall* *performance in a variety of situations?* With this goal as a foundation, the team is able to maintain focus on the individual. We can begin to look critically at the nature and extent of services that need to be offered.

Where do we want him/her to go? *What long-term outcomes are wanted for the child?* We want children with impairments to achieve their maximum potential. Treatment planners need to ask themselves if the services they are offering will help the student participate in social-interactive activities with family and friends, succeed in school, and be prepared for work and adult responsibilities. All persons who have a stake in the child's success need to participate in this discussion and believe that desired outcomes are only achievable if there is a high degree of involvement.

When do we want the child to get there? *What is the time line for implementing the program and achieving the desired outcomes?* It is important to recognize that treatment for individuals with TBI is not just something that happens and then is finished. This means that there must be continuous evaluation of the individual's performance, the strategies implemented, the people involved, and the desired outcomes. Because there is constant transition from one situation to the next, there is always a need to rethink and replan. Rather than view the child as "treated" and "cured," it is wiser to continually refocus efforts and strive for continuous improvement in performance.

Who do we want/need to take with us? *To plan and implement the program effectively, who needs to be involved?* We need to involve those individuals who hold the highest stake in the child's successes. The persons selected to participate need to have understanding of the child's strengths and needs, the policies that will have an effect on school placement and programming, the challenges the child is likely to face, and resources available for support. Whenever planning is undertaken, there should be representation from the child's family, school, community, and the disciplines offering services.

How do we want to go? *What approaches to treatment are most effective for meeting the needs of youngsters with TBI?* Any mode of treatment that will bring about the desired outcomes should be tried. Thus, innovative thinking and continually seeking opportunities to improve the process are two important planning concepts. Much of the fun of using this philosophical approach comes from creating or trying new approaches designed for other types of populations or applying approaches from different disciplines. It is essential to build on an individual's existing strengths rather than focus on correcting behaviors or weaknesses.

In this model, the child is not the only person targeted for improvement of skills or acquisition of important change strategies. All team members need to be a part of the learning process: gaining a better understanding of TBI, learning to work effectively together, identifying opportunities to promote the child's success, and continually striving to improve the quality of the child's performance.

How much will the trip cost—what resources will be necessary to implement the plan? *What is it going to take to achieve the desired objectives and where will the resources be obtained?* Adequate resources must be tapped to meet the child's needs. Resources include not only finances, but also personnel, time, and service options. Teaching family members to identify and access resources will strengthen programming.

How will we know when we have arrived? *What are the benchmarks against which we can measure our success?* The treatment program needs to include ongoing evaluation to determine its appropriateness and suitability for meeting a child's and family's needs. This is especially important because children with TBI experience frequent changes and transitions throughout their development. Helping a child and family to achieve a better quality of life than would have been possible without the intervention is a good mark of success.

Key Components of Proactive Planning

Following is an explanation of several key components representative of quality improvement and strategic planning processes and a brief explanation of how these concepts apply to treatment planning for youth with TBI.

Clear Vision

Plans are strengthened if they are guided by a jointly shared vision for the future for the youngster. Collaborating to develop a single, clear vision about what is possible in the future enables the team to direct energies. Visions usually are an expression of hope and are generated from the heart. By creating a positive image of the future, long-term, sustained action can be fostered. For example: The child will enjoy an independent, happy and productive life among family and friends. When creating a vision, planners need to change the mental model of the child currently held by the team. They need to think about what is possible. Only then can change in behaviors occur. Clinging to limited mental models of a child and what may or may not be possible limits planners to acting and thinking only in familiar patterns.

Of course, the vision also must be reality-based and take into consideration the complications and constraints that are likely to be confronted.

Mission Statement

The mission statement specifies how the vision will be accomplished. The mission statement provides a foundation for constancy of purpose toward which all treatment efforts can be directed. Specific planning emanates from the mission statement. An example mission statement for youth with TBI is: *to improve the child's potential for succeeding in home, school, work, and community activities by expanding opportunities and continually improving performance.*

Environment Scan and Analysis

The potential success of a child's reintegration into home, school, work, and community and subsequent transitions through life's milestones will depend on creating a favorable environment for implementation. It is important to begin the process by scanning and analyzing important environmental factors to gain needed information for treatment planning. This helps to identify obstacles that might interfere with success and opportunities that will enable it. Efforts such as these will lead to the development of strategies for dealing with factors that may hamper achievement or progress. Such efforts will also enable planners to take advantage of situations that can enhance success.

By conducting an environmental analysis, one can determine if there are policy, social, technological, demographic, psychological, or interpersonal factors that will affect the implementation of service plans. Information for an environmental analysis can be obtained through a variety of scanning techniques including observation, interactions with people in a child's life (clinicians, teachers, friends, family, co-workers), written reports about the child, review of school materials, and needs assessment tools.

Trend Analysis

The future of any endeavor is affected by trends that have an impact on it. A number of trends can have an impact on service delivery in educational settings for individuals with disabilities (Hales & Carlson, 1992). As schooling is such an important aspect of the reintegration process for children, these trends will need to be taken into consideration when planning programs for children with TBI. Hales and Carlson summarize four major trends. First, because of a critical shortage of special education personnel, additional personnel will need to acquire the skills necessary to serve students. This will blur the borderline between special education and regular education. Children with TBI will be more likely to be served within the regular education classroom versus special education classes. Second, the type, quantity, and variety of services children will need to continue to expand. This expansion will drain resources. Professionals should explore mechanisms and funds for accessing needed services. Third, desired outcomes will become more functionally-based. Therefore, programming will have to demonstrate efficacy and clearly show how students will be prepared for the challenges they face. Last, persons with disabilities will experience fewer limitations because advances in technology will enable greater access. This means treatment time should be devoted to introducing clients who demonstrate substantial disabilities to technology. Proficient use of available equipment should be encouraged. Many of the same trends are relevant in health care and rehabilitation settings. Several recommendations for working with youngsters with TBI emerge from these trends. The recommendations are presented in Figure 2–1.

Obstacles or Challenges Assessment

The trends described above, situations that occur in the child's life, and people the child encounters often pose **opportunities** for or **threats to** goal achievement. It is important to identify those trends, environmental, and interactional factors that may have either positive or negative impact on the youngster.

Over 5 years (from 1986 to 1991), we questioned health care and education professionals about their observations of problems individuals with TBI encountered during the reintegration process. In addition, we observed numerous school reentries. This yielded anecdotal information and written questionnaire responses from more than 1,500 professionals. Five barriers to successful reintegration were consistently identified as posing problems for program development, treatment implementation, and reintegration into home, school, work, and community (Blosser & DePompei, 1991). They include:

1. The impairments resulting from the TBI and the impact of those impairments on learning and social capabilities (cognitive-communicative impairments were cited as posing the most difficulty).

2. Lack of organizational readiness and capability for providing comprehensive services to youngsters and families.

3. Inadequate communication among professionals (health care, rehabilitation, education), family members, and community support systems as children moved from acute care the school setting.

4. Lack of professional understanding and preparation for meeting the needs of this group of youngsters.

1. Assessment should be functionally-based and result in an authentic assessment of abilities;
2. Instruction should occur in naturalistic settings with individualized instructional objectives and include goals directed toward the student's interests and desires;
3. Family needs to play significant roles in decision making and program implementation;
4. Alternative sources of funding will need to be sought;
5. Multiple agencies in the child's community should be involved in program implementation and services should be coordinated and shared;
6. Children with disabilities should be served within the general classroom and inclusive schools;
7. Personnel serving children with disabilities will need to expand skills, collaborate, and share responsibilities;
8. Legislation and policy changes will need to occur to better meet the needs of children;
9. Services for children with disabilities should become the joint responsibility of special and regular educators;
10. The search for effective and cost efficient services should continue;
11. Professionals delivering services will have to become more accountable for the quality of service delivery;
12. Practitioners and persons, in general, should demonstrate greater sensitivity to specific learning and interpersonal styles of children with disabilities from diverse cultural, racial, linguistic, and ethnic backgrounds;
13. Greater emphasis in programming for children should be placed on transition from school to work.

Figure 2–1. Recommendations based on current health care and education trends.

5. Family and peers' lack of understanding of the nature and implications of the disability and lack of preparation for assuming meaningful roles in developing and implementing treatment plans; lack of awareness of the rehabilitation and education processes.

For some professionals, these issues might seem overwhelming, causing frustration because they interfere with success. In assuming a proactive, strategic stance, however, these factors can be viewed as **challenges** rather than obstacles. Opportunities are sought out. Threats are recognized, confronted, and met. Treatment planning and goal setting are planned with the challenges in mind. A course of action that leads to desired results can be charted.

Planning Assumptions

These are the parameters within which the treatment plan must operate. All planning must take into consideration the positive and negative realities that will have an impact on the decisions that are made. For individuals with TBI, this would include factors such as the degree of physical wellness the child has achieved, the severity of the impairments resulting from the TBI, family resources, availability of services, and teachers' capability and willingness to help.

The treatment approach we suggest is based on several assumptions. When being reintegrated into life activities, individuals must be able to move to and function within a variety of situations and environments and with a variety of communication partners. The treatment program should be dynamic, with ongoing evaluation of its effectiveness and modification as indicated. Other persons in a student's environment have usable knowledge about the individual's needs and can contribute to planning and implementing a program. The student's communication partners can play significant roles in the entire rehabilitation process. The treatment strategies selected should be relevant to the student's needs, communication situations to be encountered, and communication partners' competency for implementing them within their environmental setting.

Goals or Program Directions That Flow From the Mission Statement

This step involves determining and prioritizing the goals to be accomplished, with consideration of the trends, planning assumptions, opportunities, and threats. Planning discussions should focus on specific, anticipated learner outcomes, teaching orientations, performance criteria and expectations for various situations, strategies others can use to improve performance, materials and modifications that should be incorporated into programming, and the like. Example goals emphasizing functional outcomes might include: *participating in social activities within the school or community, learning study skills to promote better understanding of information presented in textbooks, or taking part in home and family responsibilities.* Once the team agrees on the strategic issues of importance and the priority assigned to each, all members need to work toward achieving the same goals.

Objectives

Goals are translated into specific objectives appropriately designed for an individual. Example objectives that would correspond to the above goals might include: *participating in a minimum of two social activities per month with peers at school, understanding the rules of a game, or learning sarcastic expressions used by peers during play; identifying main topics in book chapters, answering questions at the end of a chapter, highlighting key vocabulary words; or completing two chores at home each day.*

Strategies for Achieving Objectives

A number of routes can be taken to achieve objectives. This step helps identify individuals in the child's life who are most relevant, specifying the role each person will play, the type of information that needs to be conveyed, the resources to be used, and how resources will be allocated. Planning needs to focus on developing effective skills in others.

Evaluation of Outcomes

For continued relevancy, programs must be subject to modification, as the original assumptions that guided planning may change. It is necessary to move from periodic evaluation of the youngster's capability to continuous evaluation of performance and to stimulate continuous improvement in performance.

Proactive Planning: Four Major Phases

The proactive planning process consists of four distinct and interdependent phases (see Figure 2–2). The phases can occur either independently or simultaneously. In this way, the entire planning process is viewed as continuous, with all phases related to one another. No single phase represents the beginning or ending of the planning cycle. Change that occurs in one phase will produce related changes in another. For **all** phases, there needs to be joint collaboration between professionals and important persons in the child's life.

In Phase I, the **pre-planning phase,** groundwork for planning is put into place. A design for treatment is developed. Initial team members are identified, the team is formed, and each member works to gather several pieces of pertinent data including: the student's history and current status, the environments in which reintegration will take place, and the skills and needs of people in those environments and their potential for contributing to treatment success. It is at this point that people

Evaluate

- Interweave implementation strategies into all interactions, learning, working, and playing situations
- Maintain ongoing observation
- Reassess only if necessary
- Continuously gather information from people in the youngster's environment
- Collaborate to determine need for program revision

Preplan

- Form interprofessional and interagency networks
- Collaborate with family and significant professionals
- Obtain medical and educational histories
- Assess performance
- Clearly describe behaviors (strengths, needs)
- Analyze demands, expectations in various environments, situations
- Observe performance in various contexts
- Assess capabilities of the environment (staff, competencies, resources, motivation)
- Analyze modifications necessary
- Prepare staff and others in environment to understand, problem-solve, and assist

Implement

- Take action on plans
- Observe youngster's behaviors, performance, and responses
- Associate findings with impairments
- Self-evaluate interactions, behaviors, use of strategies and procedures
- Supplement instructional materials with additional resources and technology

Plan

- Gather and collate information from family, teachers, rehab professionals, specialists, health care providers, and administrators
- Discuss history
- Describe current status
- Summarize anticipated demands and potential problems
- Indicate expectations, fears
- Explore strengths and talents
- Identify needs and recommendations of modifications
- Brainstorm an ideal plan

Figure 2–2. Proactive planning process. Planning and program revision for individuals with TBI should occur on a continuous basis. Such an ongoing, proactive planning process will foster changes in service delivery to accommodate the youngster's needs as changes occur in the youngster's skills, the environment, or demands and expectations of particular situations encountered.

begin to develop "ownership" of the proposed plan. If ownership is absent, the treatment program is not likely to be implemented.

A number of creative assessment procedures can be used to gather the desired information. This phase enables the planning team to contribute information from a wide range of perspectives. During this phase, the team identifies important questions that need to be answered about a child's characteristics and the services needed. Those questions form a framework for planning. The team will then be able to form assumptions on which planning will need to be based. It also makes it possible to identify situations that might pose obstacles or challenges to meeting goals or implementing planned actions.

During Phase II, the **planning phase**, the team begins to work collaboratively to analyze information gleaned during the preplanning phase. Then together, the team determines the youngster's strengths and needs, goals, objectives, and workable strategies for preparing the youngster to function effectively in the various environments to which the individual will return. Time is spent deciding the who, what, where, when, why, and how aspects of the treatment plan.

In Phase III, the **implementation phase**, action is taken on plans made. The climate for dynamic intervention is established and opportunities for learning are provided. This includes learning by the child, learning by professionals, and learning by family members and friends.

Phase IV, the **evaluation and improvement phase**, permits review of how the plan is working, including the goal and strategy selection. The degree of success at achieving desired outcomes is determined. The team subjects the plan to modification as new information is learned and planning assumptions change. During this phase, decisions are made regarding continuation, modification, or elimination of goals and strategies. New goals are developed in response to situations that occur as the student makes transitions.

Following planning processes such as these enables planners to approach intervention in a very systematic way. As a child progresses from the hospital through rehabilitation into school and in various transitional situations, the planning process can be maintained on a continuous basis. This will support ongoing program maintenance and improvement.

The remaining chapters of this book provide practitioners with insights for using this type of proactive planning process to serve the needs of youth with TBI.

Summary Guidelines

1. Treatment is more effective if friends, relatives, teachers, and professionals work together in a systematic way.

2. Transferring the responsibility and strategies for treatment from professionals to people who are important in the child's life requires adopting a proactive philosophical approach to planning and treatment.

3. Three key aspects of proactive planning and treatment are: (1) identifying, anticipating and responding to, or preventing problems before they increase in complexity and greatly affect the youngster's performance; (2) exercising creativity, flexibility, and ingenuity in program development; and 3) promoting teamwork and a high level of mutual involvement in planning and implementing the program.

4. The systematic steps involved in proactive planning include: establishing a clear vision, developing a mission, scanning and analyzing the environment, understanding how trends can affect service delivery, confronting obstacles and challenges, and establishing and prioritizing goals, planning strategies, evaluating outcomes and modifying treatment accordingly.

5. When treatment planning and implementation are carried out in a continuous manner, the team can respond more in a proactive manner, thus avoiding decreased effectiveness or interrupted services.

References

Blosser, J., & DePompei, R. (1991). Preparing education professionals for meeting the needs of students with traumatic brain injury. *Journal of Head Trauma Rehabilitation*, 6(1), 73-82.

Hales, R. M., & Carlson, L. B. (1992). *Issues and trends in special education*. Federal Resource Center for Special Education. Human Development Institute. The University of Kentucky.

Kreutzer, J. S., & Wehman, P. H. (1991). *Cognitive rehabilitation for persons with traumatic brain injury*. Baltimore: Paul H. Brookes Publishing Co.

Ylvisaker, M. (1993). *Assessment and treatment of traumatic brain injury with school age children and adults*. Buffalo: EDUCOM.

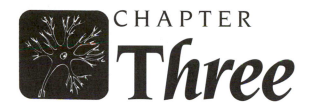

CHAPTER
Three

Working With Others

Effective collaboration and communication among family and professionals and among professionals within and between service providing facilities is needed for maximum understanding about a youngster's strengths and needs. Often, lack of communication results in loss of effective planning time, inappropriate educational placement, interrupted programming, and inadequate rehabilitative and educational services.

A proactive approach reinforces the importance of working closely with other persons who are involved in the lives, education, and intervention of youth with TBI. To productively implement this approach, it is necessary to understand the potential roles and responsibilities of family members, administrators, educators, rehabilitation professionals, and peers who directly interact with the child and can influence the effectiveness of treatment. In other words, what can we hope to accomplish by working with various individuals and how can we increase their competence for helping the child? It is also helpful to understand problems that interfere with interactions between the individual with TBI and other people and to identify tactics for forming meaningful working relationships.

Within this framework, the size, composition, goals, and function of the "team" will be continually changing as the child changes and moves through various transitions. With the child as a central focus of planning and problem solving, each team member can share their own unique expertise and contributions. Professionals and family members need to spend time together discussing ways they can best combine their talents, expertise, and schedules to facilitate a comprehensive, coordinated program for a child. Suggestions made during the discussions should be recorded in writing and incorporated into a treatment plan.

This chapter will:

1. Examine the roles, responsibilities, and working relationships we can establish with other individuals who are involved with students with TBI.

2. Determine the strategies they can use to foster improved performance by the child.

3. Discuss methods for informing others about their role and shared teaching strategies.

Meeting Friends on the Yellow Brick Road: The Importance of Collaborating and Consulting With Others

In every situation and environment a youngster enters there are demands and expectations for communication. Therefore, individuals with whom children interact need to understand the importance of cognitive communication for success. They must learn to recognize when and how disabilities are interfering with successful performance and they must implement strategies that will support or modify a child's performance. Collaborative relationships with others can be used to:

- Define and clarify the child's problems using mutually agreeable terminology;
- Generate solutions and analyze effectiveness;
- Determine the child's cognitive-communicative skills following the TBI;
- Share responsibilities for assessing and treating the child;
- Assess the impact of the cognitive-communicative disabilities on the youth's academic, social, and interactive performance;
- Define a student's communicative needs for specific educational and social situations;
- Observe a child's communicative abilities under specific circumstances;
- Develop strategies for stabilizing new skills the child is learning in therapy or the classroom; and
- Monitor the child's progress after dismissal from direct service programs.

Composition of the Team

Regardless of the medical, health care, rehabilitation, or educational setting, the preferred approach for assessment and treatment is a collaborative team approach with representation from diverse disciplines and perspectives. This collaborative model facilitates information gathering from multiple sources, broad-range problem identification, comparison of observations and perceptions, development of creative intervention approaches tailored to a child's needs, understanding of treatment approaches followed by others, exchange of roles and responsibilities, and increased opportunities to coordinate treatment efforts. As a child moves through various settings and encounters difficult situations and transitions, numerous professionals will become involved in the provision of services. Because of the nature of TBI and the resulting needs, a nucleus group of individuals should be on the team. First and foremost, family members must be involved. At least three other disciplines are fundamental: a medical professional (physician, nurse, etc.) to contribute information about the child's medical needs; an educational professional (regular and special education teacher, psychologist) to present information about the school curriculum, educational goals, and program options; and appropriate rehabilitation professionals (speech-language pathologist (SLP), physical therapist (PT), occupational therapist (OT), etc.) to describe how the child's specific impairments may affect learning and interactions and to suggest ways to implement positive change. Additionally, other professionals will become involved on an "as needed" basis to complement and enhance the quality of team efforts. Other individuals may include administrators, social workers, counselors, aides, tutors, support groups, case managers, relatives, friends, resource specialists, and others.

The second family meeting was held. This meeting included 11 people from the hospital team, my husband, and me. (Jason's Mom)

Recently, some school districts have organized **intervention assistance teams** to provide collaborative problem solving when a student performs below expectation (Ohio Department of Special Education, 1991). This is a very proactive service delivery model. Children experiencing difficulty are referred to the team for study and discussion. The team gathers information and reflects on the child's problems and needs as situations happen rather than waiting for failure to occur. Instead of one teacher trying to independently determine a course of action, a team of skilled and interested individuals works together to review information presented about a child and recommend assessment procedures and intervention strategies. The team jointly generates numerous solutions, strategies, and resources. Team members agree to undertake and share responsibilities and adhere to specified guidelines for implementing procedures and reviewing progress.

Providing this high level of support to a child experiencing problems inevitably will promote future success. Several advantages are realized from applying this model to the needs of children with TBI. It provides a forum for planning a structured approach to assessing a child and planning treatment. Inappropriate class placements will be avoided. There will be an arena for coordinating intervention strategies among multiple service providers. The child can be included and/or maintained in the regular classroom rather than pulled out into special classes. Teachers will feel supported in their efforts to teach this child with unique needs rather than afraid that they are not prepared to do an adequate job. Smooth transitions from grade to grade and teacher to teacher will be promoted, as more and more people engage in problem solving on behalf of this child. In addition, all intervention assistance team members who serve on a team for a child with TBI will have the added benefits of increasing their knowledge base about TBI, having a broader view of the students' educational needs, and learning about ways other professionals approach intervention.

Networking with Others to Develop Ongoing Effective Programming

Every treatment plan for children must reinforce the importance and need for collaboration by specifically addressing how collaborative efforts will be fostered and executed. The plans should be expressed in writing and agreed on by all parties. Two types of collaboration must take place. The first is cooperative planning and intervention among team members at the treatment facility or school. The second is forming active relationships with family and other resource persons the child might come in contact with.

Several topics should be considered when planning comprehensive treatment programming including: (a) establishing and maintaining frequent communication with family members and between professionals; (b) determining ways to access necessary and available services; (c) developing ongoing mechanisms for sharing ideas as the child progresses through key transitions and encounters situations that may pose difficulties. Because school reintegration is an important transition for children who have sustained a TBI, it is important that networks be formed between health care and rehabilitation agencies and school systems.

Developing Necessary Attitudes, Knowledge, and Skills

The attitudes others reveal about the child with TBI are crucial to the success of interactions and programming. Equally important are the attitudes professionals display toward one another and toward family members. Attitudes influence an individual's willingness and motivation to play a meaningful role in planning and implementing treatment. The actions displayed by professionals and family members are frequently directly related to their attitudes. Often, attitudes and expectations about the characteristics and behavioral patterns associated with TBI inhibit a person's ability to fully participate and contribute in helping. For example, many people have heard that individuals with TBI "don't respond to behavioral modification techniques." Therefore, they don't consider selecting behavioral change strategies in response to a child's inappropriate behavioral patterns. In fact, whether or not a child can respond to behavioral modification techniques depends more on the extent and nature of the injury, the resulting cognitive-communicative impairments, and the skill used when implementing the strategies.

Poor attitudes are sometimes the result of fear of the unknown or lack of knowledge. People have varying degrees of understanding about the nature and needs of children with TBI and the role they should be playing. Although one person cannot change another's attitude, it is possible to shape another's attitude by developing a working relationship with them and providing them with support and education. The diversity and complexity of issues surrounding TBI require a knowledge of brain injury as well as the clinical management options for delivering services effectively.

Shaping attitudes by increasing the knowledge base are only two aspects of preparing others to work effectively with a child. To make treatment effective, they need to develop appropriate skills to apply the knowledge learned. Throughout the rehabilitative and reintegration processes, crucial elements of knowledge and skills need to be learned by the family and professionals.

When recommending collaborative arrangements as part of a treatment plan, it is critical to consider the attitudes, knowledge, and skills necessary for success. The plan should reflect who the target collaborators (learners) ought to be, the content that would be helpful, the need and rationale for selection of collaborators and content, and strategies for accomplishing the training. Appendix A details many of the special competencies that should be developed by education and rehabilitation personnel who work with pediatric TBI (Blosser & DePompei, 1991;

DePompei & Blosser, 1993). These competencies can be used to plan in-service training programs as well as for selection criteria for determination of a professional's qualification to provide appropriate services.

Working With Family

Throughout this book, references are made about the importance of working with families. Family response is an important determinant of outcome for children who experience problems. Comprehensive services to children with TBI cannot be achieved without working collaboratively with the family. Family is the constant in a youth's life. They bear the responsibility for making decisions that will affect the child's life and education. Professionals simply pass through, making whatever impact and contributions they can along the way. Therefore, identifying roles and goals for family is extremely important. All plans that are developed for the child should be in conjunction with family members.

It had been a month since the accident. In my mind, the scheduling of the first family conference had taken too long. Thank goodness I have been insistent in being there, one step ahead. More communication and better education should start sooner with the parents. One person needs to focus on the parents. There were too many different people, each trying to do their own part. (Jason's Mom)

A Frightening New World for Families

The world of assessment and treatment is new and often perplexing. Before conducting assessments, time should be taken to provide in-depth explanations of the assessment about to be conducted. Rogers (1986) encourages teams to explain **why** the assessment is needed, **who** will conduct the assessment, **where** and **when** it will occur, **what kinds** of instruments or procedures will be used, and **expected outcomes** of the assessment. Additionally, family members need to understand **how** the results will be used. This will increase the family's capability to make decisions about their child and decrease anxiety. Using this approach, family members can act as resources and provide supportive information such as helping prepare the child for the testing experience, alert the tester to special circumstances, and supplement the test findings with observations about behaviors not evaluated or observed by the tester.

Although interacting with families is not new for most professionals, the importance of developing working relationships and transferring valuable information and strategies cannot be emphasized enough. The idea of incorporating persons who are significant to the child into the treatment program is based on two major premises. First, individuals can only improve their skills and develop new skills if they are stimulated to do so during the many and varied interactive situations in which they must function daily. Second, persons in the child's environment are eager and able to assist in the treatment process, but must be shown clearly how they can do so. Children with TBI often have difficulty generalizing skills from one situation to another. Progress is often slow and tedious. To foster generalization, stimulation and practice need to be carried out frequently throughout the day in natural contexts. Clinicians are unable to devote the time needed to carry out such a program of continuous practice. However, the clinician can serve as a facilitator to modify the communicative environments the child enters and teach others to interact more meaningfully and effectively. One caution is appropriate here: Care should be taken to prevent family members from becoming so eager to help that their assistance overshadows all of their interactions with the child. It is more reasonable to help them understand how to integrate their assistance into such everyday activities as home routines, meals, grooming, play, chores, and family outings.

Hints for Actively Involving Families

Based on their work with family of infants and toddlers with developmental disabilities, Winton (1990), Crais (1991), and Urbano (1992) suggest observing several underlying principles when integrating families into the intervention process. The principles apply to families of children with TBI as well:

- Treat family as equal partners in the assessment, planning, and intervention processes;
- Design services to foster the family's decision-making skills while protecting their rights and wishes;
- Encourage family members to express their joys, fears, concerns, and ideas about their child's disabilities and needs—listen attentively and respond meaningfully to what they say;
- Recognize the individuality and variability in families and modify services to meet unique needs, degrees of involvement, and styles of interaction;
- Recognize the family's strengths and needs, as well as their goals and priorities—incorporate the information gleaned into the service plan;
- Provide complete information to families, using terminology that is easily understood;

- Deliver services following coordinated and "normalized" approaches;
- Assist families in accessing support networks; and,
- Build sufficient time to work with families into treatment programs.

Family members can provide insightful information about a child's performance within the home situation, including the impact of the disability on interactions and performance of home activities. Parents are especially astute about factors that may be contributing to the child's problems and promote or hinder progress. Including family members as equal partners on the team enables opportunities to observe all team members' interactions with the student and to learn from one another.

Preparing Family To Meet Challenges

Family members (and friends) need to be prepared for the challenges that confront them when their loved one has a TBI. Professionals who are working with the child can do this as a part of the overall intervention plan. The type of information needed and the depth and amount each can learn at any given time is dependent on a number of individually based factors such as: the relationship of the family member with the person providing the information, the importance or sensitivity of the topics discussed, the timing of the delivery, the mode used for delivering the information, and the family members' receptiveness and capability of understanding and using the information. Ideally, a family will develop several competencies enabling them to meaningfully participate in planning and implementing assessment and treatment. These are:

- To understand and interpret medical and clinical reports about the nature, extent, and impact of the child's TBI and resulting disabilities;
- To demonstrate a working knowledge of all rehabilitation and educational programs in which the youngster is enrolled;
- To predict problems prior to occurrence or to identify problems as they occur and to suggest multiple strategies that might be initiated to remedy problems;
- To develop an awareness and inventory of resources that can be shared with others as the child progresses through transitional situations.

Information can be relayed to a family throughout hospitalization, rehabilitation, and reintegration. The interchange should be conducted in an organized and thoughtful manner. At all levels, an important aspect of program planning for a child is how information will be conveyed, who provides the information, and what information is delivered. These decisions should be discussed within planning meetings.

Encourage the family to keep a daily log of the child's progress and their questions for the medical and professionals who are involved. (Jason's Mom)

Family members need to be especially well prepared for their roles as **equal** team members in planning school reintegration and service delivery. Recent trends in special education and changes in federal laws encourage family members to assume more meaningful roles in not only the planning but also the implementation of educational programming for their children. Families may help set the tone and climate for establishing partnerships with professionals by informing staff of their desire to participate in the spirit of cooperation and collaboration rather than in an adversarial manner.

In school planning meetings, families should expect educators to supply test results and recommendations for class placement, academic modifications, and ideas of appropriate instructional strategies. It is important for professionals to help family members understand the pivotal role they can play in planning for effective programming for their child. Families should prepare for meetings in advance just as the education team does. They can prepare by gathering pertinent information about their child based on medical records, educational history prior to the injury, and rehabilitation reports from speech-language pathologists, occupational therapists, and physical therapists. It is also wise for family members to prepare a list of observations, interactions, experiences, intuitions, expectations, and goals for their child.

Family members will represent their child's interests better if they are prepared to discuss several key topics. They need to be provided with skills that will enable them to increase other team members' understanding of TBI and the child. They should go to a meeting prepared to explain the extent of their child's injury, the child's current status (medical, social, behavioral, and cognitive-communicative), residual strengths and weaknesses, and the functional skill areas that are impaired and how those can be expected to affect learning performance. Oftentimes rehabilitation professionals write reports indicating the extent of a child's impairments without applying the deficits to an educational setting. The family members' needs are best served if they are prepared to discuss the implications of a child's disability. Professionals can help do this by providing the family with clear examples of how a youngster might function in a classroom situation considering the specific deficits demonstrated. For example, instead of reporting that a child has **slow processing**

time, families best join the team as equal members by explaining that **a child may need extra time to complete homework assignments or to answer a question in class because of slowed information processing abilities.** Cohen's (1991) illustration of the kind of information most relevant to family members and educators alike is presented in Figure 3–1, which translates deficits to educational behaviors.

Family members should be given the opportunity to express their anxieties and concerns regarding the youngster's school placement, academic program, and therapy services. Their agenda for topics to be discussed during planning meetings might include: the family's highest expectation for the child, ideas for how personnel and educational programming appropriate for the youngster's needs might be selected, descriptions of their

Cognitive impairment	Resulting behavior
Poor attention or concentration	Distractibility: fragmented understanding of tasks; problems completing work
Poor orientation to place, person	Confusion: trouble getting around class and building, following schedules, and connecting places, people, materials with activities
Poor retention and retrieval of information	Uncertainty about what is known or has been learned
Impulsivity	Problems with attending, processing information, staying on task, and social interactions; tendency to get into situations where physical safety is compromised
Overload (comprehension breakdown)	Confusion, stress; shuts down when tasks are too long or too complex
Poor organization of thoughts, expression, tasks	Problems with comprehension, reasoning, problem solving, spoken/written expression, and task completion; difficulty planning activities during free, unstructured periods
Poor initiation	Inability to keep up with class; confusion and frustration because others view inactivity as resistance or inability to perform
Slow processing and performing	Poor comprehension of class material; cannot get work done on time
Inflexibility	Resistance, confusion, stress when confronted with changes in activities or variables in reasoning and problem-solving tasks
Inability to think or perform independently	Inability to do tasks that are expected in classrooms
Inability to generalize	Problems connecting old and new information or seeing patterns in processes; need for teacher assistance and cuing to continue learning; cannot learn or work independently as others do
Denial/poor awareness	No recognition that abilities have changed; resistance to participating in new programs; wants to return to premorbid class

Figure 3–1. Impact of cognitive impairments on learning experiences.

perception of how the youngster has changed as a result of the TBI, the family's level of understanding about how educational organizations and systems work, contributions the family is capable of making in implementing the educational plan, other family problems or preexisting situations that may affect the child or the family's participation, and ideas regarding the type and degree of supportive services needed to help their child achieve the highest potential.

Family and professionals should share ideas with one another regarding resources and teaching strategies that may help the child. In addition, it is beneficial for family to receive a clear understanding of the structure of their local school district, the district's capabilities for providing needed services, and the procedures they should follow for making inquiries, expressing needs, and accessing services. Families cannot be expected to participate equally in the reintegration process without such information.

Treatment plans should specify (in writing) ways in which family can be encouraged to take leading roles in planning and implementing services for their children. Needless to say, everything that is explained to family should be presented in a spoken or written format that is understandable. This means using simple, straightforward terminology. The explanation should be presented in a relaxed, distraction-free environment and in an unrushed timeframe.

Individualized Family/Peer Intervention Plans

A number of formats can be used for presenting important information to others. The selected format should be well suited to a family's lifestyle and cultural needs. The individualized family/peer intervention plan (IF/PIP) shown in Figure 3–2 is designed as a mechanism for facilitating discussion of the roles family members and friends can play in treatment, treatment strategies they can implement, and preparation that may be needed for full family participation. Use also assures that planners determine the instructional formats to be used for conveying the information and resources that family and friends will likely need.

Collaboration Among Facility-Based Team Members: Harder Than It Looks

Collaboration begins at home. A mutual problem-solving orientation toward assessment, treatment planning, and service delivery facilitates common goal setting and responsibility sharing among all disciplines within a facility. To implement an approach such as this, each team

Individualized Family/Peer Intervention Plan
(IF/PIP)

Name _____

Address _____

Phone _____

Parent/Guardian _____

I. Individuals To Be Involved.

Create a list of key individuals with whom the child interacts. The list may include family, friends, peers, teachers, co-
workers, neighbors and so on. Determinants for inclusion on
the list would be relationship to the child; willingness to participate; opportunities for interaction; awareness of the influence of his or her own communication manner or style
on the child; awareness of the child's TBI, strengths, needs,
and so on; ability to learn to apply treatment strategies.

II. Specific Topics To Be Discussed For Meaningful Assistance To Occur

There will be great variability in each person's level of understanding depending on several factors, including the information they have learned since the youngster was injured,
how and when the information was presented, and the manner in which it was presented. There may be gaps in knowledge that will need to be addressed. Discussion of the
following topics would increase understanding: type and extent of injury; important medical implications and course of
treatment; resulting impairments; impact of impairments on
performance, interactions, and relationships; management
methods and techniques; resources; and educational/voca-
tional considerations.

III. Presentation of Critical Information to Promote Involvement and Problems That May Interfere With Involvement

Because of the complexity of information to be presented and
laypersons' varying capabilities for absorbing difficult mate-

rial, information should be delivered over an extended time from the onset of the injury and throughout rehabilitation and school reintegration. The professional discipline of the messenger is not as important as the substance, accuracy, and timing of the message delivery. The barriers to conveying necessary information and implementing a collaborative partnership should be identified, clarified, and discussed openly at this point in the planning process. Examples might include competing commitments, restricted funding, conflicting schedules, lack of motivation or interest, fears, lack of awareness, cultural differences, diverse levels of knowledge and expertise, and counterproductive attitudes or feelings.

IV. **Instructional Formats To Be Used and Timing of Presentations**

It is not realistic to believe that clinicians will be able to conduct face-to-face in-servicing with all of the persons who are significant in a child's life. Therefore, creative and resourceful methods need to be tried for transmitting important information. Adults learn via numerous methods. Teaching formats that can be used include formal and informal meetings, audio- and videorecordings, lectures, telephone exchanges, role playing, written materials, newsletters, question-answer exchanges, support groups, group discussions, demonstrations, and observations. Those that can be most appropriately matched to the key person and topics to be discussed should be selected. The timing for discussing complex information and making recommendations is critical. The family must have reached a point where they are "ready" to hear and use specific types of information.

V. **Important Environmental and Communication Characteristics To Be Considered**

Each participant must learn to recognize the influence environmental factors and communicative characteristics have on the child's performance; how they contribute to problems and how they can influence positive change. Prior to recommending that a significant treatment strategy be imple-

Figure 3–1. Individualized Family/Peer Intervention Plan. (*continues*)

mented, the environment and communication behaviors of the key people should be analyzed and discussed.

VI. **Selection of Appropriate Goals, Targets, and Priorities for Treatment. Specific Actions To Be Taken (by Whom, When, How). Specific Time Lines.**

Those goals and objectives that will lead to the greatest potential success for the child should be selected as targets. Because laypersons will just be learning how to participate, the target goals should be limited to just a few. Examples include: helping the youngster formulate questions, redirect attention, decrease negative behaviors, organize thoughts, follow written instructions.

VII. **Indicate the Specific Strategies, Techniques, and Resources To Be Used. Provide Supportive Guidance.**

Based on the child's unique problems, strengths, and needs, key people should be taught to identify elements of the environment that are limiting the student from achieving successful experiences (with the above target skills, for example) or are posing barriers to success, elicit specific types of communication behaviors, correct errors, and seize opportunities for assisting, alter the environment, and modify their own communication style in response to the child's actions. Factors such as these should be established as target goals and objectives for the participant to learn. Teach others to monitor patterns of behavior, seize opportunities to help, and make adjustments in their own interactions that will improve performance potential. Match the strategy to meet the child's needs as well as the partner's capability. Simplify the partner's role so it will be doable.

VIII. **Evaluation and Quality Improvement**

As each segment of the program is implemented, the success and benefits should be analyzed and evaluated. Changes should be made when necessary to bring about improvement in quality of service delivery. In addition, as the child grows, changes, and transitions through various phases and situations, modifications will be needed to maintain appropriate programming.

Figure 3–2. (continued)

member (including the family) has to be willing to work with other team members to jointly establish and address priority outcomes for the child.

Different facilities use different models for team intervention. There are three major models: (1) multidisciplinary, (2) interdisciplinary, and (3) transdisciplinary. Haynes, Moran, and Pindzola (1990) present an excellent discussion of these models, how they differ from one another, and how each is utilized in the school setting. These models can be viewed on a continuum of cooperation and communication among team members, with the transdisciplinary model representing more coordinated group cooperation in planning and implementation, as well as greater communication. The transdisciplinary model provides an excellent format for promoting the type of interactions and planning this book details. In the transdisciplinary model, a child's outcomes are incorporated into daily routines and all team members contribute to the development of the assessment and treatment options. The consultation level is high during the assessment period, with all team members observing, evaluating, collecting data, and forming impressions about the child. Team members strive to work across discipline boundaries for most effective intervention.

Two of the primary stumbling blocks in achieving facility-based communication and collaboration are unclear communication and "territorialism." These factors are counterproductive to effective service delivery. Each discipline has a number of professional terms and modes of approaching and treating specific disability categories. To collaborate, all team members have to strive for better understanding of what each does and the unique way each approaches clients. They then need to be willing to exchange information and share roles. In this model, it makes no difference if a child achieves an outcome when working with the SLP, OT, or PT. The critical goal is correction of the problems and progress by the youngster with TBI. This means changing attitudes, increasing knowledge bases, and exchanging skills as in the example:

> A child who displays a communication deficit reducing the youngster's ability to process information effectively and efficiently, may not be able to follow instructions presented by the occupational therapist or physical therapist during sessions. The therapist's first inclination might be to assume that the child is operating at a lower level and reduce the task presented. In fact, the communication problems may be limiting the child's abilities to perform the task. All team therapists need to develop a clear understanding of how the communication deficit affects the child's performance in their treatments. This information can be presented by the speech-language clinician during a PT or OT session. The other therapists then need to understand and learn to use interactive communication skills to promote more efficient information processing (presenting

instructions at a slower rate, presenting instructions in smaller chunks, using more demonstration to model the performance task). In such ways, the potential success of all therapies will be increased. In addition, it is more likely that skills targeted in one treatment situation will be generalized to others.

Interagency Collaboration and Communication: Making Connections

Children with TBI proceed through numerous transitions as they stabilize medically; progress through rehabilitation, re-establish home, school, work, and community routines; and mature. It is often the exception rather than the rule that transitions are well planned and executed. Unfortunately, the lack of communication networks and protocols for exchanging information between people who play key roles as the child is transitioning results in interrupted or ineffective service delivery. Several recommendations for promoting interagency collaboration and communication are presented in Table 3–1.

Working With Educators

The classroom teacher is the individual most responsible for implementing a youngster's educational program and monitoring academic performance. The teacher can contribute information about learning objectives, curriculum, and teaching techniques generally used to present information to students. In addition, the teacher also can answer questions about events that occur within the classroom.

Educators sometimes express fears about teaching children/adolescents with TBI. This leads to decreased self-confidence in the educator's ability to provide a meaningful learning experience for the child. The lack of confidence might be perceived by the teacher, family members, or other professionals who have worked with the child and feel "ownership" in the program.

Educators' fears may be based on a number of real or imagined .factors. The primary basis for fear is lack of knowledge and understanding of the learning characteristics, problems, and needs this group demonstrates. Myths about how youngsters with TBI do or do not respond to specific instructional strategies create doubt in some educators about a youngster's ability to benefit from placement in their class. In addition, many teachers express concern about the possible extra efforts they believe they must expend in working with the child with TBI in compari-

***Table* 3–1.** Recommendations for promoting interagency collaboration and communication.

Recommendations for Promoting Interagency Collaboration and Communication
1. Identify transitions that may create obstacles for the child.
2. Inform family and persons who will be involved in the transition of the potential problems the child may encounter and recommended solutions *early*, preferably *before* the transition takes place and the problems occur. For example, for school age children, it is wise to initiate contact with the school district as soon as the injury occurs and the child is medically stable, so arrangements can be made for identifying people on each respective staff to be liaisons between agencies.
3. Exchange information that will lead to effective planning. Examples of topics that should be addressed include: the nature and implications of the TBI; the child's history (medical, school, rehabilitation, social); methods to be used for gathering and exchanging information about the child's strengths and limitations; the expectations, demands, and requirements of the transitional environment; predictions of potential problems the child will encounter; and knowledge and skill base of persons the child will encounter in the receiving transitional setting.
4. Develop an understanding about the organizational system; laws, policies, and procedures that pertain to this student; and the personnel and resources available in the transitional setting.
5. Implement an information exchange via the liaisons and face-to-face meetings to promote better understanding of the responsibilities of the sending and receiving transitional settings to clarify for each the necessary steps to take to prepare for the child's transition. For the child returning to the school setting, this means discussion of professional preparation, laws and policies that will affect service delivery, admission/eligibility criteria, placement, curriculum, and the like.
6. Develop procedures to reinforce ongoing communication after the transition has been initiated for continued development of positive attitudes, increased awareness and understanding, and treatment skills.

son to other children in their class. Some fear they do not have the competence to teach these children, because of gaps in their own training background and previous teaching experiences. Teachers' reluctance is not unreasonable, considering the number of years many may have spent perfecting their craft. Some educators may have experiences with children with TBI that were unpleasant or unsatisfying. Many educators are "comfortable" with their traditional teaching style and believe changes can interfere with their capabilities to be effective or successful.

Regardless of the cause for confidence loss or who may not have confidence in an educator's ability, the situation creates a risk that the instruction will not be successful or effective. A better and proactive plan is to prepare a teacher and classroom learning situation in **advance** of a student's arrival in class. This can be done by enhancing the teacher's knowledge and understanding of TBI and identifying applicable and appropriate teaching strategies already in the teacher's instructional repertoire. These steps result in important benefits by instilling the teacher confidence needed to implement the best educational program for all students.

Collaborative Training and Development

To promote the kind of service delivery, interactions, collaborative arrangements, and effective transitions discussed here, all individuals involved must be appropriately prepared. Professionals, as well as family members and friends, are likely to feel overwhelmed by challenges that accompany living, teaching, working, and playing with a child with TBI. Comprehensive training and development of individuals who will play significant roles in the child's life is needed.

When planning team training and development programs, it is essential to consider the audience characteristics, competencies, and roles they will be playing. There should be an interdisciplinary emphasis, clarifying each discipline's perspective and also recognizing overlap of competencies and how collaboration can take place. Perhaps the most critical aspect of any programming is to recognize the skills and competencies the audience brings to the training program. Preparation efforts are maximized if individuals can generalize what they already know about serving other populations to working with youngsters with TBI. Professionals enter the process with a broad base knowledge of instructional methods and procedures. They need simply to learn how and when to apply what they already know.

How Do We Teach Adults New Tricks?

We live in a busy and complex world. It is frequently difficult to coordinate and conduct training and development programs. Constraints such as limited funding, restricted time, conflicting schedules, and competing professional commitments pose obstacles. As solutions to these obstacles, program planners should use alternative approaches to conducting training. First and foremost, it is important to remember that the audience comprises adults who respond to a variety of teaching methods. This means that "adult-learning" options varying from the traditional seminar and lecture format can be used to provide the training. Several adult learning options that have been employed successfully are presented in Table 3–2.

Table 3–2. Adult learning options.

---
* Audio- or videotape presentations
* Informal discussion and question-answer groups
* Panel discussions
* Self-study programs
* Meetings focused on solving a particular problem

Training and development programs offer opportunities for disseminating valuable information to others. Learning can be conducted over an extended time, thus enabling learners to better absorb the information rather than ingest it rapidly and become overwhelmed. Unless a concerted effort is made to provide all team members with the skills and competencies they need to be effective partners, participation will be limited and gains made by the individual with TBI will be stifled. Durgin, Schmidt, and Fryer (1993) compiled an extensive resource of content and process suggestions for developing staff skills to meet the needs of individuals with TBI. They discuss principles and methods of staff development, preparation of staff for clinical intervention, and management issues related to staff development. Several sections of their resource are particularly helpful for structuring training and development programs targeted on ethical issues related to service provision to this population and specific clinical intervention strategies. Areas include family-centered rehabilitation, development of a positive communication culture, behavior analysis, implementation of supported employment services, staff needs for employees in residential settings, sexuality issues, medical perspectives, and substance use.

Summary Guidelines

1. Collaboration and communication must take place between family and professionals and among professionals to promote understanding about the individual's strengths and needs.

2. The size, composition, goals, and function of the team will continually change as the youngster changes and develops.

3. Recommendations regarding the role team members can play should be based on the demands and expectations for communication in specific situations and environments.

4. Interactions and transitions will be most successful if aspects such as positive attitudes, knowledge about TBI, and skills for helping are in place.

5. The participation of family members and educators in the treatment program is very critical for children/adolescents with TBI.

6. Professionals can contribute much to developing the understanding and competencies of people who are significant in the lives of youngsters with TBI.

7. Efforts to involve family members and other individuals will be more successful if a plan is thoroughly conceptualized and developed.

8. Many formats may be used to promote effective training and development programs for professionals and family members.

References

Blosser, J., & DePompei, R. (1991). Preparing education professionals for meeting the needs of students with traumatic brain injury. In R. DePompei & J. Blosser (Eds.), School reentry following head injury. [Special issue]. *The Journal of Head Trauma Rehabilitation, 6*(1), 73–82.

Cohen, S. (1991). Adapting educational programs for students with head injuries. In R. DePompei & J. Blosser (Eds.), School reentry following head injury. [Special issue]. *Journal of Head Trauma Rehabilitation, 6*(1), 56–63.

Crais, E. R. (1991). Moving from "parent involvement" to family-centered services. *American Journal of Speech-Language Pathology*, 5–8.

DePompei, R., & Blosser, J. (1993). Professional training and development for pediatric rehabilitation. In C. J. Durgin, N. D. Schmidt, & L. J. Fryer (Eds.), *Staff development and clinical intervention in brain injury rehabilitation* (pp. 229–254). Gaithersburg, MD: Aspen Publishers, Inc.

Durgin, C. J., Schmidt, N. D., & Fryer, L. J. (1993). *Staff development and clinical intervention in brain injury rehabilitation.* Gaithersburg, MD: Aspen Publishers, Inc.

Haynes, W. O., Moran, M. J., & Pindzola, R. H. (1990). *Communication disorders in the classroom.* Dubuque, IO: Kendall/Hunt Publishing Company.

Monsen, R. (1986). Phases in the caring relationship: From adversary to ally to coordinator. *Maternal Child Nursing, 11*, 316–318.

Ohio Department of Education, Division of Special Education, Statewide Language Task Force. (1991). *Ohio handbook for the identification, evaluation, and placement of children with language problems.* Columbus, OH: Ohio Department of Education.

Rogers, S. J. (1986). Assessment of infants and preschoolers with low-incidence handicaps. In P. J. Lazarus & S. S. Strichart (Eds.), *Psychoeducational evaluation of children and adolescents with low-incidence handicaps.* New York: Grune & Stratton.

Urbano, M. T. (1992). *Preschool children with special health care needs.* San Diego: Singular Publishing Group, Inc.

Winton, P. (1990). A systematic approach to inservice training related to P.L. 99-457. *Infants and Young Children, 3,* 51–60.

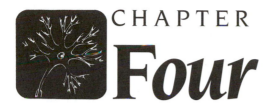

CHAPTER

Four

Transition Issues and Quality of Life Outcomes

The Individuals with Disabilities Education Act of 1990 (IDEA) specifies that **transition plans** be provided for all students with disabilities. The intent of this portion of the law is to prepare students to make the transition from school to work. Wehman (1992), provides a traditionally accepted definition of transitions, suggesting that they are "the life changes, adjustments, and cumulative experiences that occur in the lives of young adults as they move from school environments to more independent living and work environments." He explains that transitions include "changes in self awareness, body, sexuality, work and financial needs, and the need for independence in travel and mobility" (p. 5).

This view of transitioning may be rather limited because it is focused only on transition from school to work. In reality, individuals with TBI are continually confronted with transitions—from situation to situation, setting to setting, and communicative interaction to communicative interaction. Transitions occur when a child/adolescent moves from the medical setting to rehabilitation center and from there to home care. Within rehabilitation programs, transitions occur as a child moves from therapy to therapy. As medical and physical improvements are made, a child gains greater independence and moves from the home setting to school and community activities. A child is constantly confronted with transitions from informal, comfortable situations in the home to more formal, structured situations in the school and community. In school, transitions take place on an ongoing basis, as the child changes subjects, classrooms, buildings, teachers, study groups and so on. Each transition can pose difficulty and stress for all parties concerned — the client, the family, and the professionals who provide services. All of this places the concept of transition in a broader sense.

Another major milestone. Jason came home for a day. Thank goodness I have been a step ahead along the way; otherwise, I would have panicked at the thought of him coming home so soon. I rented a beeper which was to be my communication device between the hospital, doctors, therapists, anyone who was connected to Jason's recovery. I found the beeper to be the most valuable source of communication to bring my son back. I had been learning all along how to care for him. (Jason's Mom)

Transition into each situation carries with it unique and different demands and expectations for performance. To succeed during each transition, it is incumbent on the child/adolescent to make adjustments. Some of the adjustments that are necessary are very apparent. Many more are subtle and require skilled observation and response. It is important to recognize and identify the problems that youngsters encounter during transitions and to develop functional strategies to improve response and performance. In addition, people in the child's life can learn to recognize the obstacles posed during transitional situations and facilitate change in features in the environment or modify their own behavior to provide better support for the child.

This chapter prepares readers to:

1. Recognize the commonalities of transitional situations confronted by individuals with TBI.
2. Identify factors that influence transitions.
3. Describe several principles that underlie transition planning.
4. Follow suggested guidelines for developing an effective transition plan.
5. Understand the importance of helping individuals achieve quality of life outcomes.

Factors That Influence Transitions

Transitions are affected by many influences. These may include: (1) the extent of the impairments resulting from the TBI; (2) the demands and expectations of specific situations; (3) the level of understanding and re-sponsiveness of people to the individual's behaviors; (4) quality of treatment services provided to the student and his or her family; (5) opportunities to succeed made available to the student; and (6) the readiness, preparation, and motivation exhibited by the student and his or her family. For a youngster to progress through multiple transitions successfully, changes must occur in the child, in the people the youngster will encounter, in the services that support the transition, and in the opportunities offered. The assessment process should be designed to determine the modifications to provide the most support for the child in transitional situations.

Current literature about transitioning for populations with disabilities reinforces consideration of aspects such as student choice, family choice, and self-determination in transition planning (Rosenkoetter, 1992; Wehman, 1992). With this viewpoint, the control for making decisions regarding goals and needs rests with the person with the disability and his or her family, rather than with service providers. This is a much more proactive and client-focused approach. For this to take place, transition planning should help the client participate in meaningful activities. Social networks should be developed and expanded and recreational opportunities offered. For some, technological advances will enable successful transitioning.

Planning Transitions

To prepare youngsters for multiple transition experiences, treatment needs to include preparation in prerequisite skills as well as on-site skill development. Perhaps the most important prerequisite skill for any transition is the ability to communicate within that environment and situation. Processes should be implemented for ongoing identification of problems prior to their occurrence. The child and family must be provided with strategies for confronting problems before they become insurmountable. The relevance and importance of treatment plans and objectives in relation to transitions must be considered.

Given these thoughts about transition planning, several principles for planning transitions (regardless of the type of transition) can be identified (see Table 4–1).

Guidelines for Transitional Programming

Following are several guidelines to assist in the implementation of transitional programming:

Table 4–1. Principles for planning transitions.

Principle I:
The child and family members must be included as equal partners in planning transitions.

> Unless input is sought from those who are to be involved in the transition, planning efforts may be futile and useless. The treatment strategies to be implemented will be more likely to be understood and carried out if considered to be valuable and important.

Principle II:
Prerequisite skills that will be necessary for success during the transition should be the focus of treatment and intervention.

> The behaviors that should be targeted for change and development should be based on the identified skills the child will need to function within the transitional situation or setting.

Principle III:
Emphasis should be placed on preparing the transitional environment and people in the environment to support the youngster and help facilitate successful performance.

> Professionals should devote work toward identifying and modifying those features of the transitional environment that might pose challenges or obstacles for the child. In addition, the quality and quantity of support and resources available should be increased. Similarly, family members, friends, and others can take very active roles to ensure smooth transitions.

Principle IV:
The results of the transition should be evaluated to determine future directions.

> The outcome of the participation in the transitional experience should be a sense of accomplishment, success, confidence, and competence on the part of the youngster as well as others who provided support.

1. Include the child and family in transition planning efforts; seek their input and value their contributions. Prepare the family for their role in transition planning by providing them with needed information and skills to participate meaningfully. Encourage them to share information, establish priorities, set goals, and make decisions. Teach them to evaluate their own understanding, coping skills, strengths, functioning style, needs, priorities, and resources.

2. Involve other important individuals who might provide insights about transitional situations and be able to provide assistance to the child through the transition.

3. Provide students with options and opportunities to participate in multiple community experiences.

4. After age 14, include vocational assessment (formal as well as informal) as part of a multifactored evaluation process. Use the information obtained in the development of individualized transitional services indicated on the student's treatment plan.

5. State the numerous types of transitions the youngster will likely encounter. Indicate them on the intervention plan (individual family service plan, individual education program, individualized transition plan and so on.)

6. Develop a multiyear plan for preparing the student for transitioning, considering the student's preferences, needs, interests, and potential in light of the obstacles that may be encountered. Take steps to ensure that the child gains the skills necessary to succeed.

7. Specify (in writing) the persons who will monitor the delivery of services to prepare the student for transitions.

8. Establish interagency collaborative agreements to identify services available, services needed, and to develop an action plan to deliver transitional services. Create a service system without gaps and interruptions in service delivery. Facilitate transmission of important information. (Rosenkoetter [1992] refers to this as a "seamless" service system.) Representatives from agencies that deal with vocational education and rehabilitation, mental health, health and human services, postsecondary education, adult education, trade schools, and other appropriate agencies should be included.

9. Involve administrators and policy makers, specifying how transition planning will be incorporated into the systems of the sending and receiving agencies, how families can be involved, and how critical documents (treatment plans, IEPs, IFSPs, etc.) will be in place at the beginning of the transition. Clarify the roles and responsibilities of each party, funding needed to make the transition work, and program evaluation issues.

10. Spend time and resources preparing staff to participate in training to increase their understanding of systematic transition planning.

11. Prepare the environment for the youngster by removing obstacles to facilitate full inclusion and participation.

Quality of Life Outcomes

Discussion in recent special education literature reinforces the use of "quality of life" as a context for planning and evaluating services for groups of individuals with disabilities (Dennis, Williams, Giangreco, & Cloninger, 1993; Halpern, 1993). In service delivery programming for TBI, this is reflected in efforts to prepare individuals for effective participation in home, school, work, and community activities. Recent legislation and evolving professional practices support this philosophy.

Universal agreement does not exist on the definition of quality of life, specific methods for identifying quality of life indicators, or procedures for determining if quality of life outcomes have been achieved. Goode (1990) provides us with the following definition that can be used operationally to help improve our understanding of this concept:

> When an individual, with or without disabilities, is able to meet important needs in major life settings (work, school, home, community) while also satisfying the normative expectations that others hold for him or her in those settings, he or she is more likely to experience high quality of life. (p. 46)

Of course, those aspects that represent quality of life for one person may differ greatly from those of another. To pursue a quality of life framework, personal needs and perspectives as well as societal perspectives and expectations must be recognized. Practitioners should maintain an open attitude about what might represent quality of life for persons with TBI and their families, showing respect for diversity in beliefs and values (Dennis et al., 1993).

Edgar (1987) provides a list of what he regards as minimal entitlement for quality of life. His list includes: safety, pleasantness, friends and companions, self-esteem, fun, accomplishments/productivity, and excitement. Although others may generate completely different lists, this one exemplifies the types of quality of life aspects that should be taken into consideration when making a long-range plan for education and/or intervention services. Using quality of life as a planning springboard, individuals and family can be encouraged to express their personal goals for intervention. Agencies and organizations can strive to develop programs and policies that address the perceived transitional needs of those they serve (Halpern, 1993). The quality of life objectives established can be used to monitor the student's progress and make modifications in intervention and teaching to ensure that successful outcomes are achieved.

Halpern (1993) offers the following list of outcomes that might be used to structure and evaluate transition programs:

I. Physical and material well-being
   - Physical and mental health
   - Food, clothing, and lodging

- Financial security
- Safety from harm

II. Performance of adult roles

- Mobility and community access (e.g. uses some form of transportation effectively)
- Vocation, career, and employment (e.g. has a job reflecting career interest)
- Leisure and recreation (e.g. uses free time to pursue interests)
- Personal relationships and social networks (e.g. maintains positive involvement with friends)
- Educational attainment (e.g. earns a high school diploma)
- Spiritual fulfillment (e.g. participates in spiritual activities of choice)
- Citizenship (e.g. votes)
- Social responsibility (e.g., doesn't break laws)

III. Personal fulfillment

- Happiness
- Satisfaction
- A sense of general well-being

Benchmarks for Making Decisions

Transitional and quality of life issues should form the basis for assessment and treatment planning. Each assessment procedure that is selected and goal that is developed should be measured against these two issues. Will the assessment procedure selected provide the type of information necessary to adequately prepare the child to function as the individual progresses through numerous and various transitions? Will the goals established for treatment lead to successful transitions and ultimately a better quality of life for the child? Will the treatment approaches implemented prepare not only the child for what is ahead but also the environment he or she is to enter and the people within that environment for their roles?

Summary Guidelines

1. Transition planning is mandated by federal and state legislation for providing services to individuals with disabilities, including those who have sustained a traumatic brain injury.

2. Transition must be viewed from a broad perspective.

3. Transitions are influenced by numerous factors and these factors must be considered when planning treatment.

4. Preparation in prerequisite skills as well as on-site skill development are important aspects for transition planning.

5. Following suggested principles and guidelines for transition planning will assist team members in developing individualized transition plans tailored to the individual's needs.

6. Quality of life outcomes can be used as a context for planning and evaluating services.

References

Dennis, R. E., Williams, W., Giangreco, M. F., & Cloninger, C. J. (1993). Quality of life as a context for planning and evaluation of services for people with disabilities. *Exceptional Children, 59*(6), 499–512.

Edgar, E. (1987). Early morning thoughts on the quality of life. Unpublished manuscript. University of Washington, Seattle. In A. S. Halpern, (1993). Quality of life as a conceptual framework for evaluating transition outcomes. *Exceptional Children, 59*(6), 486–498.

Goode, D. (1990). Thinking about and discussing quality of life. In R. Schalock & M. Begab (Eds.), *Quality of life: Perspectives and issues* (pp. 41–58). Washington, DC: American Association of Mental Retardation.

Halpern, A. S. (1993). Quality of life as a conceptual framework for evaluating transition outcomes. *Exceptional Children, 59*(6), 486–498.

Rosenkoetter, S. E. (1992). Guidelines from recent legislation to structure transition planning. *Infants and Young Children. 5*(1), 21–27.

Wehman, P. (1992). *Life beyond the classroom: Transition strategies for young people with disabilities.* Baltimore, MD: Paul H. Brooks Publishing Co.

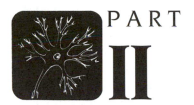

PART

II

Assessment of Cognitive-Communicative Strengths and Needs: A Problem-Solving Approach

If the only tool you have is a hammer, you tend to treat everything as if it were a nail.

(Author Unknown)

Assessment for children/adolescents with TBI is not an easy matter. A variety of possible impairments that influence behaviors, a number of functional situations that elicit different types of responses, and a number of persons will affect communication abilities. The tools for assessment must be as unique, varied, and individualized as the child. Otherwise, we may as well employ the same tool (routine standardized test protocol) regardless of the type of nail before us!

A proactive approach to assessment of cognitive-communicative impairments requires a perspective that subscribes to three interrelated aspects of communication: (a) Describing the demands of the environment, (b) Knowing the capabilities of the person with TBI, and (c) Defining the capacity of persons in the environment to play meaningful roles by understanding their impact on the person with TBI and altering the manner and style of communication interactions with and demands on the individual with TBI accordingly. Figure II–1 is a model of that concept.

Cognitive-Communicative Performance Capabilities in Specific Situations

After determining the demands and expectations of a communication situation (Figure II–1, #1), the ability of the person to adapt to the contexts must be examined. For example, if an individual is unable to maintain a topic in a group discussion and has problems formulating answers to questions, reorienting to the topic or proposing alternative means of responding may be necessary. Informal observation or simulation of situations allows the clinician to propose workable solutions to the problems a youngster is likely to encounter. By fitting a person's skill levels to the demands of the situation, acceptable alternatives can be developed.

Demands and Expectations Requiring Communication

The cognitive-communicative skills a person needs to perform successfully in most situations (Figure II-1, #2) can be identified. For example, most teachers require a student to answer questions verbally during discussion groups; workers in a job setting are expected to be able to engage in shoptalk as well as chitchat; family members are expected to participate in dinnertime conversations and complete daily chores. Assessing the specific expectations and demands of likely situations for a particular child/adolescent contributes much to the treatment planning process.

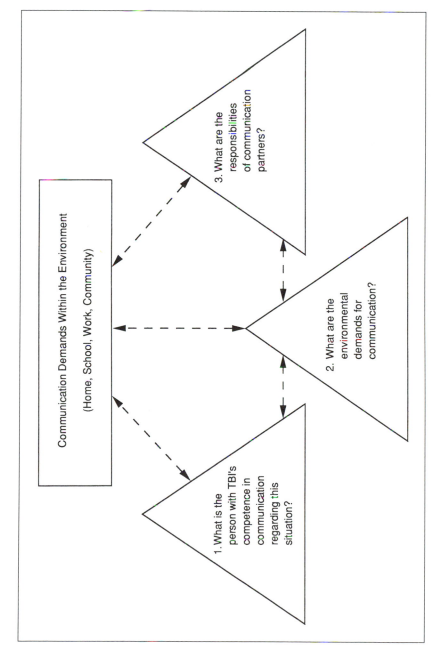

Figure II–1. Interrelated aspects of communication.

Communication Demands Within the Environment

(Home, School, Work, Community)

1. What is the person with TBI's competence in communication regarding this situation?

2. What are the environmental demands for communication?

3. What are the responsibilities of communication partners?

Communication Behaviors of Others

It is important to analyze other communicators in the environment to determine their style of interaction with the individual in treatment (Figure II-1, #3). The quality and effect of others' verbal and nonverbal responses during various interactions with the child/adolescent, and their ability to modify communication efforts to facilitate improved responses should be noted.

When all three aspects are considered part of the assessment process, the most descriptive and useful information can be obtained and applied for treatment in all environments of the child/adolescent.

Part II familiarizes professionals with a variety of methods and techniques to be employed to assess various aspects of communication important to the child/adolescent with TBI. Readers should be able to:

1. Describe general considerations for assessment of the child/adolescent.

2. Outline an assessment plan that includes both formal and informal assessment procedures based on the present performance of the child/adolescent with TBI.

3. Develop a problem-solving technique that guides structure of the assessment so it will be the most beneficial process for the person with TBI.

4. Understand procedures for evaluating the demands and expectations of the cognitive-communication environment.

5. Suggest methods for understanding the communication partner's impact and responsibilities in the communication interaction.

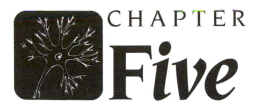

CHAPTER

Five

Understanding Individual Cognitive-Communicative Capabilities

The child/adolescent with TBI has been described as an individual who will continue to change as the youngster develops. This development alters behaviors, strengths, and needs. If the child/adolescent is considered to be a changing, developing person, a one-time diagnostic assessment and creation of an intervention plan based on that assessment may not be the most reliable means of understanding cognitive-communicative functioning. Assessment might be better viewed as an ongoing, interactive process. Comprehensive programming should regard evaluation for the child/adolescent as always changing and based on the desire for both formal and informal assessment of capabilities and needs of the individual as the child develops over time.

To adequately assess, it is necessary to understand some general considerations, review both formal and informal procedures, and develop a proactive problem-solving system that suggests what evaluation procedures may be useful.

What Should An Evaluator Think About? General Considerations for Assessment

Assessment techniques are employed to screen, diagnose, evaluate for placement, garner baseline performances, plan ongoing treatment, monitor treatment progress, and make discharge decisions. This chapter is based on the concept that ongoing goals of assessment should be to (a) provide updated and complete description of capabilities and needs that the person exhibits, (b) apply the child/adolescent's cognitive-communicative strengths to support new or relearning situations, and (c) suggest areas for remediation of cognitive-communicative needs through treatment that is directed toward the best possible reintegration to functional situations within home, school, community, and work.

DePompei and Blosser (1993) outline a number of relevant issues relating to assessment that should be emphasized. These include:

1. **Medical history.** Children may have reasons other than the TBI for impairments they exhibit. Information regarding any prior conditions that may have contributed to impaired cognitive-communicative skills should be obtained from all possible sources. Possible confounding conditions include developmental delays, neurological disorders, medical conditions, abuse, and previous illnesses.

2. **Developmental history.** Information regarding developmental milestones achieved prior to the TBI is useful in determining whether or not other physical, cognitive, communicative, behavioral problems may have existed prior to injury.

3. **Effects of medication on performance.** Many youth will be taking antiseizure or other medications. Knowledge about the medication prescribed and possible effects on test and treatment performance is essential.

4. **Educational and work history.** Knowledge of the type of student or worker this individual was before injury is essential for determining potential after injury. It is possible that the person had problems with learning prior to the injury and an inability to perform in school is not related to the TBI, but to preexisting abilities, attitudes, or interests.

5. **Test environment.** Optimal results are obtained in a quiet, one-on-one test environment. But results may not reflect or predict a child's performance in functional situations with many distractions. Therefore, additional observations in real-life situations are helpful.

6. **Timing of the assessment.** Telzrow (1991) suggests that assessments should not be given to children/adolescents during periods of rapid

growth or recovery. When the child/adolescent is rehearsing new learning or has plateaued may be the best time for formalized evaluation.

7. **Redundancy across agencies.** When discharge from one facility takes
   place, another agency often begins services for a given child/ado-
   lescent. To meet each facilities' entrance-exit criteria, assessment
   often takes place on both discharge and admission. Agencies should
   work together to jointly determine tests to be given and the appropriate facility to conduct assessment. This will result in findings that
   are more relevant for treatment and placement in the new facility,
   elimination of duplication of testing, more effective use of families'
   and professionals' time, and reduced costs.

8. **Recognition of strengths of the individual.** Professionals are trained
   to recognize impairments in individuals and to help compensate for
   them. It is essential that the strengths also be documented. Statements about strengths in the assessment reports are useful when
   planning treatment and reintegration strategies.

For a while there, everyone was so willing to emphasize Jason's negative points and it was time to remind them of his positive attributes
as well. I asked his teachers if they had said "great job Jason" to him
lately. They both admitted they had not, and followed through with
my suggestion which made Jason feel good. (Jason's Mom)

---

9. **Involvement of family members.** Family members can often provide important clues as to how an individual can be motivated and
   assessed. Obtaining their insight prior to and throughout assessment
   and treatment is important.

10. **Use of consumer advocates.** Oftentimes, agencies cannot or should
    not advocate for specific programming or assessment at another fa-
    cility. There are consumer advocates for children, such as the Coa-
    lition for Handicapped Children, who will provide impartial third
    parties to assure the best possible services for children/adolescents.
    They should be regarded as friends and used to help facilitate as-
    sessments, planning for transitions, and implementation of treatment
    programs. Figure 5–1 provides a format for including these impor-
    tant issues in an assessment protocol.

Being Proactive Counts: Planning for Assessment

Assessment should emphasize the importance of formal and informal
evaluation of strengths and needs of the child/adolescent and how these
will affect reintegration. All types of assessment provide valuable infor-

IMPORTANT CONSIDERATIONS FOR ASSESSMENT

_____ 1. Is there anything about the child's medical history prior to the injury that should be considered when preparing for assessment?

Medical Problems:

Surgery:

Medications:

_____ 2. What is the medical history relating to the TBI?

Physical Problems:

Cognitive-Communicative Problems:

Medications:

Other of Significance:

_____ 3. Is there prior educational history of special classes or services provided?

_____ 4. What is the developmental history prior to injury?

_____ **5.** What is the prior work history?

_____ **6.** What agencies have been involved to date?

   Facility
      Length of time in facility:
      Services offered in facility:
      Tests administered and results:

_____ **7.** What strengths are noted?

   In agency reports:

   In family reports:

_____ **8.** What was the family told about:

   previous assessments:
   functioning levels:
   transitioning:
   TBI:
   support groups:

_____ **9.** What information can the family provide regarding:

   learning styles:
   hobbies, interests:
   food, music, clothing likes:
   personality:
   discipline procedures and responsiveness to them?

_____ **10.** Are there people who can serve as local supports or resources in transitioning or assessments?

Figure **5–1.** General considerations for assessment checklist.

mation regarding present abilities and potential for developing skills for performance in a variety of functional settings. This section discusses both formal and informal assessment techniques.

Formal Assessment

It is important when determining intervention and compensation procedures to understand all variables that contribute to the behavior that should be stimulated or altered. Standardized tests certainly contribute to the understanding of that process. Typically, assessment is regarded as selecting a standardized test and evaluating the person within the parameters of the test. Obtaining formalized empirical data about the cognitive-communicative functioning of children/adolescents with TBI is considered beneficial, as it can define how expressive and receptive language difficulties, as well as higher-order language processes, are affected. It provides information about variables of performance that is standardized and contributes to understanding of underlying cognitive-communicative processes that may be impaired. Formalized assessment is often still necessary to determine eligibility for services or placement in some agencies such as schools or mental health facilities. With increasing demands for efficacy of intervention, formalized methodologies appear to be an important means of documenting how cognitive-communicative therapy can contribute to progress and change.

Benefits of evaluation with standardized tests include:

1. Data are consistent from child to child.
2. Children/adolescents are familiar, and often comfortable with formalized tests.
3. Information can be quantified and tests can be repeated and compared.
4. Efficacy of procedures is more universally accepted among professionals when based on formal assessments.
5. Generalization of data may help professionals understand all the facets of functioning affected by the TBI.

A number of articles have been written regarding formalized assessment of individuals with TBI. For detailed information regarding test domains and specific tests that may be useful with this population, the reader is referred to articles by Begali (1987), DePompei and Blosser (1991b), Groher (1990), Kennedy and Deruyter (1991), Lehr (1990), Sohlberg and Mateer (1989), Telzrow (1987, 1991), and Ylvisaker (1985, 1993).

Few formalized tests have been normed on the population of individuals with TBI. One test which is specifically developed and normed for individuals 15 and over with TBI is the Scales of Cognitive Ability for Traumatic Brain Injury (SCATBI) by Adamovich and Henderson (1992). Additional information about application for adolescents with various problems resulting from TBI should be forthcoming as professionals around the country respond to and publish data on its use.

Although one test for adolescents 15 and older is on the market, it is important to note that standardized tests specifically designed for young children/adolescents with TBI are not available. Russell (1993) suggests this is because of the heterogeneous nature of the disorder. She further states, "Because of the variability in functioning across different settings and tasks, it is unrealistic to assume that one instrument could reliably identify the scatter of strengths and weaknesses in communicative function commonly observed after brain injury" (p. 71). It may be useful to employ a selected battery of age-appropriate tests when determining the cognitive-communicative strengths and needs of a particular child/adolescent.

Occasionally, professionals choose to employ tests that are not designed for children or adolescents. These tests may not be considered as valid descriptors of behaviors of children. Issues of developmental appropriateness are of major concern and application of obtained results is limited.

Modification of a test or subtest has become a subject for discussion in the past few years. For example, Ylvisaker (1993) and Russell and Grantham (1992) suggest that violating basals, ceilings, and time limitations may yield additional functional information about language functioning as well as demonstrate areas of preserved abilities. Some of the modifications in testing that have been suggested by DePompei and Blosser (1987), Ylvisaker (1993), and Russell (1993) include:

1. Allow untimed testing;
2. Divide testing into several sessions to allow for fatigue or loss of attention;
3. Lengthen the test time to determine if attention to task decreases or if child can persevere;
4. Introduce auditory or visual distractions such as testing in a classroom, cafeteria, or busy physical therapy area;
5. Reduce distractions to one-on-one in a quiet environment to determine maximum performance potentials;
6. Enlarge printed materials or place fewer items on each page;
7. Permit different types of response modes, such as gesturing, or writing, rather than relying on verbal responses.

8. Restate test directions by using simpler directions or by making directions more lengthy and complex.

9. Employ pictures or printed cards to reinforce understanding of test procedures;

10. Repeat and cue to determine if multiple bits of information will stimulate recall;

11. Select various subtests of different tests according to the needs of the individual;

12. Observe pragmatic language skills during testing to sense appropriate use of problem solving, questioning, turn taking, self-monitoring;

Any change in the standardized testing protocol should be documented in the report of test results. Not only will this provide greater insight into the child/adolescent's capabilities, but it may lead to techniques that can be incorporated into treatment.

Although standardized tests can provide important information about language functioning, questions about the exclusive use of standardized tests with this population have been raised.

Concerns About Use of Formalized Tests

Reliance on a battery of standardized tests that have some limitations cannot provide a full, accurate data for understanding the total communicative needs of this population. Kreutzer (1993) suggests that many persons with TBI may perform within the normal or slightly below range on standardized tests. He states that formalized tests do not always yield the lowered performance scores often required for placement. He reports that conversations with family, peers, teachers, and employers reveal that regardless of scores obtained on such tests, an individual with TBI is often not performing at normal levels in the home, school, or work situation. He questions the exclusive use of standardized tests and the usefulness of the obtained information for real-world situations.

Ylvisaker (1993), Kreutzer (1993), Russell (1993), Blosser and De-Pompei (1992), Cohen (1991), Ewing-Cobbs, Fletcher, Levin, and Landry (1985), and Baxter, Cohen, and Ylvisaker (1985) suggest that accurate description of performance potential may suffer if only formalized assessments are employed. These concerns include:

1. Testing provides estimates of optimal rather than typical levels of performance;

2. Testing in a quiet one-on-one environment can control for attention and concentration problems that may be present in natural environments;

3. Formal explanatory directions for taking the test may provide structure for recall of previously learned information that cannot be spontaneously recalled or applied outside the test situation;

4. Clarity of test directions may mask self-initiation difficulties and inability to independently shift from one task to another;

5. Structured tests may not allow for evidence of slowed processing;

6. Limited time periods allotted in assessment do not allow evaluation of ability to learn new information and retain it over time;

7. The examiner may provide structured encouragement that is atypical of other communicators in the environment. Thus, social strain and stress associated with performance in normal communication situations may be eliminated;

8. Automatic skills learned before injury are typically not forgotten and may show as automatic responses during testing;

9. Short testing segments mask problems with distractibility over time or allow for no data for persistence needed to complete a task;

10. Use of standardized basal and ceiling will not uncover gaps of information that may be lost below basal or for abilities that may be present above ceiling (characteristic of TBI).

These concerns appear to be sufficient to require additional information from other sources when assessing. Informal assessment is necessary to provide the most comprehensive picture of function. Russell (1993) suggests that assessment should be guided by "(a) questions about the student's contextual and functional use of language, and (b) questions about the impact of verbal and cognitive deficits on communicative functioning" (p. 72). Combining standardized test scores with informal observation and assessment should provide the most complete picture of the child/adolescent's functioning and potential to perform in a variety of settings.

Testing by therapists right before he was discharged showed that he was severely impaired in perceptual functions, cognitive sequencing and mental tracking, memory and learning, orientation, and attention. He was struggling with feelings of depression, sadness, anger, and frustration, which he hid beneath a facade of a lack of concern and passive acceptance. (Jason's Mom)

Informal Assessments

Informal assessment procedures provide valuable information for clinical decision making. The tests should be completed in more natural environments, such as cafeteria, classroom, or during family visits, rather than one-on-one optimal situations. These assessments can provide information about performance in real life situations.

Functional assessments offer more flexibility to the practitioner who is hoping to effect changes in the cognitive-communicative behaviors of a child/adolescent with TBI. Functional assessment denotes the observation and documentation of antecedent and consequent events that contribute to communicative behaviors with both positive and negative consequence. Determining pertinent situations that hold significance for the teacher, boss, family, or friends and aiding the child or adolescent to function adequately in those situations is the goal of functional assessment.

Carr and Durand (1985) and Day, Rea, Schlusser, Larson and Johnson (1988) indicate that there is some validity for basing treatment procedures directly on functional assessment of behaviors. Durand and Carr (1987) also call for prior functional assessment when devising procedures to reduce problem behaviors. Lennox and Miltenberger (1990) suggest that not completing a functional assessment prior to initiating treatment may present risks because (a) the client may be exposed to an ineffective treatment regimen that is counter-productive (b) effective procedures may be delayed, and (c) the treatment selected may have aversive results, not appropriate for the needs or goals of the client.

DePompei and Blosser (1991b) outline several types of informal functional assessment that may be helpful. These include direct observation, interviews and surveys, and experimental manipulation of variables believed to be related to the behavior in question.

Direct Observation

Direct observation of the child or adolescent with cognitive-communicative problems is often the most useful means to understanding what is happening within a real-world environment. Behaviors that appear to be appropriate in a one-to-one situation often are not so in a different environment. For example, a child may be able to maintain adequate attention to task in a quiet environment, but be unable to transfer that behavior to the home where many distractions in the form of TV, radio, phones, and multiple conversations interfere with maintenance of attention to the assigned task. A teenager who is very auditorially distractible reported that she was quite capable of watching a TV movie. Her mother reported this was true as long as nothing interfered, such as the phone ringing or asking if she would like a bowl of ice cream. If these distractions occurred, the teen was likely to become outraged by the distraction and would be unable to resume watching the story.

Because cognitive-communicative behaviors may be very different in the classroom, work, or home, the best means of determining the factors that may account for an alteration in performance is to spend time observing the situation and the persons found in it. When unable to place the child/adolescent in the real situation, it is also possible to observe behavior patterns among families and friends when they visit a rehabilitation facility or to simulate real world environments

Ylvisaker et al. (1990) suggest a variety of probes for exploring cognitive-communicative behaviors in children. Figure 5–2 is an adaptation (Duerk, 1990) of these behaviors that can be used as a checklist while completing direct observations.

Interviews and Surveys

Interviews and surveys are a viable means of obtaining information about a child/adolescent's cognitive-communicative behaviors. They are probably the most effective when combined with direct observations, self-monitoring, and rating scales. (Cone, 1987; O'Leary & Wilson, 1986). Interviews can be conducted with parents, peers, relatives, teachers, and staff of rehabilitation facilities to determine what the cognitive-communication behaviors were prior to the injury and what they are presently.

Development of an informational checklist that includes pertinent data that can be applied to home, school, or community according to specific needs at the time is one means of obtaining this information. Figure 5–3 (DePompei & Blosser, 1991b) is a model of one such questionnaire. It is based on information deemed necessary for development of home or school cognitive-communicative skills that would be important for acceptance by peers or family.

Self-monitoring questionnaires also can be very helpful in understanding and developing executive functioning skills in the older child or adolescent. Use of this type of survey is dependent on the cognitive-communicative abilities of the client as well as the ability to self-assess and determine personal strengths and weaknesses. Figure 5–4 is a self-monitoring questionnaire developed for an adolescent who had returned to school. Paul was having specific difficulty restraining himself from "humorous" outbursts in the classroom. Although the teacher reported that some of his speaking out was appropriate and humorous, she indicated that he had no ability to know when to stop or when he was offending classmates and the teacher. This self-monitoring questionnaire is based on work completed by Blackwood (1971). It was employed to help Paul assess his behavior. Findings then formed a basis for modifica-

Student name _____ Date of birth _____
School _____ Diagnosis _____
Classroom _____ Date _____

		Y	N
ATTENTIONAL PROCESSES	1. Can be aroused		
	2. Can maintain attention		
	# minutes during testing		
	# minutes during therapy		
	# minutes during favorite acitivity		
	3. Attention span increase:		
	when distractions are reduced		
	when task is familiar		
	when reward is offered		
	when instructed to pay attention		
	4. Can shift attention from one activity to another		
	Maintains topic appropriately		
	Shifts topic appropriately		
	Perseverates		
	Can maintain conversation while performing a motor task		
PERCEPTUAL PROCESSES	1. Eyes focus on people		
	Eyes focus on objects		
	2. Eyes track moving objects/people		
	Cross midline		
	3. Can identify familiar objects in a picture		
	Can complete a puzzle		
	Can sort objects		
	4. Matches pictures		
	Identifies object that is different		
	Completes math problems		
	5. Can find a specific item among many		
	Can find an object in a picture		
MEMORY/ LEARNING PROCESSES	1. Able to recall: events from day to day		
	locations around the building		
	2. Can answer yes/no questions: about a story told to them		
	about a story they read		

			Y	N
	3.	Can retell a story: with props		
		without props		
		with distractions		
		without distractions		
		with incentive		
		without incentive		
	4.	Can list words in a category		
	5.	Shows use of rehearsal strategy		
	6.	Asks for repetition/clarification		
ORGANIZING PROCESSES	1.	Can describe: how to play a game		
		a familiar object		
	2.	Can select materials to complete a project		
	3.	Can sequence events of the day: with cues		
		without cues		
	4.	Can construct things with building blocks		
	5.	Can answer main-idea questions		
REASONING/ PROBLEM-SOLVING PROCESSES	1.	Can sort according to a rule		
	2.	Can predict outcomes		
		Prevents negative outcomes		
	3.	Can complete if-then statements		
	4.	Completes word analogies		
	5.	Explains proverbs		
	6.	Provides several possible solutions		
	7.	Asks for help		
	8.	Keeps working		
	9.	Gives up		

Figure 5–2. Cognitive-communication observational checklist. (From DePompei, R., & Blosser, J. L. [1991b]. Functional cognitive-communicative impairments in children and adolescents: Assessment and intervention. In J. Kreutzer & P. Wehman [Eds.], *Cognitive rehabilitation for persons with traumatic brain injury: A functional approach* [pp. 226–227]. Baltimore: Paul H. Brookes Publishing. Copyright 1991 by Paul H. Brookes Publishing. Reprinted with permission.)

It is important that we understand the activities in which your child participated. This information will help us design intervention that is meaningful to your child and you. Please fill in all information as completely as possible.

1. List the names, ages, and relationship of everyone living in your home.

2. Are there other children, relatives, or individuals who previously lived in your home? Please list names, ages, and where they are now.

3. What special hobbies or interests does your child have?

4. What kind of food does your family like to eat?

5. What holidays does your family enjoy celebrating?

6. Are there any special traditions that you have when celebrating holidays or birthdays?

7. Indicate who in your family routinely completes the following tasks. Place a star on those items for which your child has been or could be responsible.

Task	Father	Mother	Child	Comments
Setting table				
Cooking meals				
Clearing table				
Washing dishes				
Grocery shopping				
Unpacking groceries				
Laundry				
Ironing				
Putting clothes away				
Sewing/mending				
Cleaning house				
Care of pet				
Emptying garbage				
Yard cleanup				
Mowing grass				
Repairs around house				
Car maintenance				
Homework				
Attendance at school activities				
Attendance at school conferences				
Other				

8. If discipline were necessary for your child, how would this be done and who would do it?

9. When there is a major family decision to be made, who makes it?

10. List activities you enjoy as a family.

100

---

11. List names and ages of your child's friends, and activities they enjoy.

    Name   Age   Activities

12. What school activities has your child enjoyed in the past?

13. Would you classify your child as outgoing or shy?

14. List any community activities in which your child participates (scouts, swimming lessons, art classes, library hour, etc.).

15. Write any additional information about your child that you think we should know.

Figure 5-3. Family information sheet. (From DePompei, R. & Blosser, J. L. [1991b]. Functional cognitive-communicative impairments in children and adolescents: Assessment and intervention. In J. Kreutzer & P. Wehman [Eds.], *Cognitive rehabilitation for persons with traumatic brain injury: A functional approach* [pp. 222–223]. Baltimore: Paul H. Brookes Publishing. Copyright 1991 by Paul H. Brookes Publishing. Reprinted with permission.)

tion, as Paul was taught to use the information obtained from the first evaluation as a baseline against which behaviors on subsequent days were measured. One peer in the class as well as the teacher also answered similar questionnaires so that Paul had additional input about his achievements in altering his behavior.

Several formalized scales evaluate problem behaviors (Lennox & Miltenberger, 1990). These scales are devised to look at problem behaviors of severely developmentally delayed individuals. But, it appears that some application might be made with children and adolescents with TBI. One formal scale is the Motivation Assessment Scale (Durand & Crimmins, 1988) which looks at how a behavioral problem is reinforced. Another by Donellan, Mirenda, Mesaros, and Fassberger (1984) is designed to determine the communicative function of problem behaviors. The various ways in which a behavior may be reinforced by the actions of another person is provided for professionals to evaluate. Adaptation of these formalized scales can provide another means of confirming the patterns of behavior and how they appear to others who are communicating with a child or adolescent with a TBI.

Experimental Manipulation of Variables

When a particular behavior is of concern, experimental manipulation of controlling variables may be helpful in completing a functional assessment. Durand and Carr (1987) outline a method of manipulating variables associated with problem behaviors in a classroom. By careful analysis

Date: _____

1. Mark the number of times you interrupted Mrs. McCann's class today.
   1 2 3 4 5 6 7 8 9 10   more than 10
2. How did Mrs. McCann respond to your interruptions?

Response	Number of times
____ She smiled and laughed	____
____ She didn't laugh	____
____ She ignored me	____
____ She talked while I was talking	____
____ She interrupted me	____
____ She told me to stop	____

3. How did the kids in the class respond?

Response	Number of times
____ Laughed	____
____ Were quiet	____
____ Looked at me funny	____
____ Told me to stop	____
____ Didn't care	____

4. What did you do wrong in Mrs. McCann's class?

5. What happens that you do not like when you speak out in Mrs. McCann's class?

6. What should you have been doing?

7. What happens that you like when you raise your hand and speak only when called on by Mrs. McCann?

Figure 5–4. Classroom monitoring form. (From DePompei, R., & Blosser, J. L. [1991b]. Functional cognitive-communicative impairments in children and adolescents: Assessment and intervention. In J. Kreutzer & P. Wehman [Eds.], *Cognitive rehabilitation for persons with traumatic brain injury: A functional approach* [p. 224]. Baltimore: Paul H. Brookes Publishing. Copyright 1991 by Paul H. Brookes Publishing. Reprinted with permission.)

of antecedent events and manipulation of variables, they were able to identify specific activities that triggered the undesirable behavior and suggest manipulations of events that might alter the behavior. Telzrow (1994) suggested a series of specific tasks to identify a problem behavior and design specific means of alteration. Figure 5–5 is an outline of her procedure.

Although many professionals who work with children and adolescents with TBI would state they do not have the time to develop such extensive procedures to evaluate behaviors, the procedures present a viable option for examining problem behaviors and suggesting alternatives for modification of behaviors. The time expended may be worth the effort, if undesirable behaviors can be modified by understanding the controlling variables and employing modifying controls.

PROBLEM-SOLVING ASSESSMENT AND INTERVENTION WORKSHEET

Student _____ Grade _____ Teacher(s) _____

Meeting Date _____   _____

Collaborators _____   _____

_____   _____

_____   _____

Step 1. Behavioral description of problem _____

_____

_____

_____

_____

Common Pitfalls	Guiding Questions
1. Concern is vague or general	• What is it you would like _____ to do to be successful? • What would it be like if the problem weren't there?
2. Description is not behavioral	• What does _____ look like?
3. Jumping to generating interventions before problem is analyzed	• Do we fully understand the problem yet?

Step 2. Behavioral statement of desired goal or outcome _____

_____

_____

_____

_____

_____

Figure 5–5. Problem-solving assessment and intervention worksheet. (From Telzrow, C. F. [1994]. Best practices in facilitating intervention adherence. In A. Thomas & J. Grimes [Eds.], *Best practice in school psychology* [3rd ed.]. Washington, DC: National Association of School Psychologists. Copyright [1994] by the National Association of School Psychologists. Reprinted by permission of the publisher.)

(continues)

Common Pitfalls	Guiding Questions
1. Goal is vague, not in behavioral terms.	• Would we have the goal if we reversed the description of the problem?
2. Stating the goal in "eliminative" or "dead person's" terms (i.e., absence of behavior).	• What are the replacement behaviors we would like to substitute for the problem behaviors?

Step 3. Analyze the problem by generating and testing hypotheses about why the behavior is occurring:

_____ occurs because _____
(Problem Behavior)   (Hypothesis)

Guiding Questions

1. Generate hypotheses in all categories:
 	
   a. Curriculum
   b. Instruction
   c. School/classroom environment
   d. Peers
   e. Home/Community
   f. Child characteristics
 	
2. Test the likelihood of each hypothesis by making prediction statements:
   If _____ , then _____ .
   (Positively phrased hypothesis)   (Desired outcome/goal)
 	
3. Determine need for collecting additional data to help analyze problem. <u>Collect only essential data.</u>
 	
4. If necessary, adjourn and reconvene after essential data are collected.

Step 4. Given hypothesized reason for problem, brainstorm possible interventions _____

_____

_____

_____

_____

_____

Common Pitfalls	Guiding Questions
1. Evaluating ideas as they are generated.	• Let's just list ideas now, and evaluate later.
2. Limiting suggestions to what is currently in place.	• If we could do anything what intervention would we design?

Step 5. Evaluate alternatives and select intervention.
        (Star alternatives above)

Common Pitfalls	Guiding Questions
1. Tendency to see a specific place or person as an intervention.	• Is that an intervention, or a place where intervention occurs?
2. Selecting interventions that are unrelated to the hypothesized reason for the problem.	• Will that intervention address the cause of the problem?
3. Giving referring teacher sole responsibility for implementing interventions.	• How can we share responsibility for implementation?

Step 6. Clarify the intervention and develop action plan, goal, monitoring procedure, and review date.

By —————————— , student will ——————————
         (Review Date)   (Behavioral Goal)

as demonstrated by ——————————————————— ,
                        (Monitoring Procedure)

as a result of this intervention: ———————————
                                    (What and how much)

to be implemented by ——————————— , ——————— .
                           (who)   (when)

Common Pitfalls	Guiding Questions
1. Failure to specify goal or review date.	• What do we expect and when do we expect it?
2. Failure to thoroughly describe intervention.	• How will ——————————— (Social skills training, etc.) be implemented?
3. Failure to incorporate monitoring procedure.	• What data will we use to evaluate the effectiveness of this intervention on the review date?

Step 7. Implement the intervention and provide for long-term carryover as necessary.

Figure 5–5. (continued)

Common Pitfalls	Guiding Questions
1. There is no commitment to implement plan (intervention) adherence)	• Problem-solve about reasons why and develop plan to address.
2. Intervention is not implemented as planned (treatment integrity)	• Provide training, guided practice.
3. Intervention is restricted to a specialized service.	• Strategy is taught to others

Step 8. Evaluate the effectiveness of the intervention and continue or revise plan as necessary.

Common Pitfalls	Guiding Questions
1. Data from monitoring procedure are not available.	• Clarify/revise monitoring procedure.

Figure 5–5. (continued)

Milton, Scaglione, Flanagan, Cox, and Rudnick (1991) outline a number of techniques for developing functional assessments based on interests and daily activities of the person with TBI. These include:

1. **Skill integration** is employing multiple behavioral domains and drawing on multidomain integration. For example, a classroom assignment to write about George Washington requires ability to recognize and understand vocabulary, extract bits of information from a resource, organize information into sequential sentences and paragraphs, employ problem-solving skills, and maintain focus even if distracted. The researchers recommend computer games such as the Carmen Sandiego series to evaluate skill integration in functional activities.

2. **Critical thinking** is evaluating information, accepting or rejecting ideas on objective grounds, raising questions about the accuracy and relevancy of information, and weighing the merits of the source of information. The researchers suggest using strategy games such as Connect Four or Othello, which require a number of higher level thought processing and reasoning skills.

3. **Visual processing** is understanding the visual processing problems including delays in interpreting what is seen. Consultation with an optometrist or ophthalmologist who has experience with TBI is recommended.

4. **Conversational processing** is comprehension of bits of auditory information as presented while screening out extraneous visual or auditory

distractors. The researchers indicate that traditional central auditory batteries may lack sensitivity to critical aspects of processing conversations of lectures. They suggest employing real-life bits of information, such as newscasts and documentaries presented in typical environments like a TV lounge area. A question-and-answer session to determine what is understood and retained can be employed immediately after viewing and following a period of time.

Additional information about informal assessment in functional situations can be found in Blosser and DePompei (1992), Kreutzer and Wehman (1991), Rosenthal, Griffeth, Bond, and Miller (1990), Williams and Kay (1990), Ylvisaker (1985, 1993), and Ylvisaker and Sezekeres (1994).

Let's Try It Another Way: Problem-Solving Assessment

Various aspects of communication will be considered by the professional who wishes to define the cognitive-communicative strengths and needs of the child/adolescent with TBI. It is apparent that information of significance can be obtained from both formal and informal assessment. Knowing when to use various assessment techniques is essential to ongoing planning.

What follows is a suggested decision-making plan that can be used to move an examiner through the assessment process. It is impossible to make this plan inclusive of all severity levels and potential implications of individual settings and task requirements. It is intended as a guide to be modified as necessary for individual persons with TBI. It is based on several aspects of communication functioning: cognitive-communicative processes of perception, attention, memory, processing speed, executive functioning, and receptive, expressive, and social pragmatic language skills. It is focused on understanding the individual's cognitive-communicative performance capabilities in specific situations.

It is suggested that assessment take place in a number of settings, such as quiet one-on-one, cafeteria, physical therapy or occupational therapy area, classroom, and so on. Both formal and informal assessment should occur in varying settings to obtain the best picture of cognitive-communicative strengths and needs within a number of contexts.

It is helpful to regard communication as a series of interdependent interactive processes. Figure 5–6 is a highly simplified interactive communication matrix that pairs various processes (speed of processing, memory, attention, executive functioning, expressive language, receptive language, pragmatic language skills) with developmental aspects, allowing the most comprehensive view of a child/adolescent.

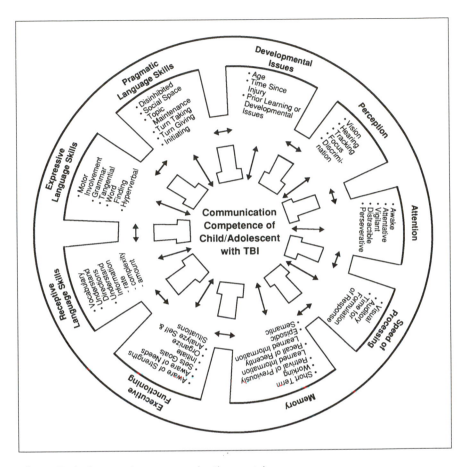

Figure 5–6. Interactive communication matrix.

With this interactive matrix in mind, and understanding that processes usually overlap, the following problem-solving approach is suggested. This approach is based on the writings of Adamovich, Henderson, and Auerbach (1985), Begali (1987), DePompei and Blosser (1991a, 1992), Gerring and Carney (1992), Groher (1990), Harrington (1990), Kennedy and Deruyter (1991), Rosen and Gerring (1986), Russell (1993), Sohlberg and Mateer (1989), Telzrow (1987, 1991, 1994), and Ylvisaker (1985, 1993). Resources for the formal tests suggested are found in Appendix B.

Initial Questions:

1. What is the real life experience for which this person is preparing or is currently participating?

2. What are the communication demands of this experience or situation?
3. How can I determine the capabilities and needs of this person in this situation?

After answering the first two questions, consider the cognitive-communicative strengths and needs from the following perspective to answer the third question.

PERCEPTION

Is there evidence of perceptual problems that will interfere with performance in communication?

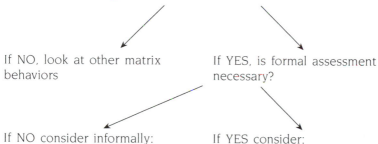

If NO, look at other matrix behaviors

If YES, is formal assessment necessary?

If NO consider informally:

1. Ability to focus visually or auditorially on pictures, objects, voices.
2. Ability to visually track across a page or among several pictures or objects.
3. Ability to visually or auditorially discriminate among pictures, sounds, objects.

If YES consider:

1. Medical evaluation to rule out vision or hearing problems.
2. Constructional Praxis Tests, such as Test of Visual Motor Skills (ages 2–13) or TVMS: upper level (ages 12–40) Psychological and Educational Publications.
3. Central auditory processing battery
4. Developmental Test of Visual Motor Integration (Follett Publishing Co.)

Is data sufficient to define strengths, needs, and direct treatment?

If NO
Consider

If YES
develop goals and initiate treatment

ATTENTION

Are there problems with impaired attention skills that will affect performance in communication?

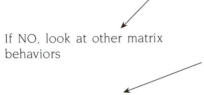

If NO, look at other matrix behaviors

If YES, is formal assessment necessary?

If NO consider informally:

1. Level of arousal: (to people, time of day, stimulus presented)
2. Vigilance: can attention be maintained to task completion?
3. Distractibility: Unable to maintain attention to task in noise, busy environment?
4. Perseveration: Unable to shift from one task to another or one topic to another?

If YES consider:

1. Attention Deficit Disorders Evaluation Scale (Hawthorne Educational Services)
2. Fisher's Auditory Problems Checklist (Life Products)
3. Wisconsin Card Sorting Test (Wells Printing Co., Inc.)

Is data sufficient to define strengths, needs, and direct treatment?

If NO
Consider

If YES
develop goals and initiate treatment

MEMORY

Is performance indicative of memory problems that will affect performance in communication?

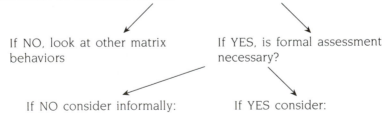

If NO, look at other matrix behaviors

If YES, is formal assessment necessary?

If NO consider informally:

1. Short term memory skills:

If YES consider:

1. Oral Commands CELF (Psychological Corporation)

a. Able to follow increasingly complex directions?
b. Able to respond to verbal or written directions one at a time, two at a time, etc.?

2. Working memory
   a. Can direction be held long enough to complete?
   b. Can piece of information (phone number, page of math assignment) be recalled long enough to complete task?
   c. What is memory span for unrelated words (numbers, random words, visual symbols)?

3. Long term memory
   a. Episodic:
      1) Can retell events of the day, week?
      2) Can recount experiences of interest (outings, parties), from past?
      3) Can recount experiences from present-new game, classroom activity, work experience?
   b. Semantic:
      1) What is retained vocabulary in conversation?
      2) Where are gaps in previously learned information?
      3) How is previously learned skill

2. Oral Commission DTLA-2 (PRO-ED)

3. Visual Auditory Subtest: Woodcock-Johnson Psychological Test Battery (R) (DLM Teaching Resources)

4. Token Test for Children (DLM Teaching Resources)

5. Digit span TOLD (PRO-ED)

6. Numbers Reversed subtest: Woodcock-Johnson Psychological Test Battery (R) (DLM Teaching Resources)

7. Denman Neuropsychology Memory Test, Denman (1984), Charleston, N.C.)

8. PPVT (R) (American Guidance Service)

9. Language Tests-TOLD (PRO-ED); CELF (The Psychological Corporation)

10. Academic achievement based on curriculum already studied

11. SAT or ACT (compare to previous scores)

12. Group achievement tests (compare to previous scores)

13. Selective Reminding Test: Woodcock-Johnson Psycho-Educational Battery (DLM Teaching Resources)

(addition, typing)
completed now?

4) How are rules for
games learned
preinjury recalled?

5) What is present
academic achieve-
ment level?

4. Retrieval

a. What is skill in
recalling information
given or activity
performed immedi-
ately vs. 1/2 hr., end
of day, next day?

b. Is ability to retrieve
information aided by
visual or auditory
cueing?

c. What is recalled
best—facts, main
idea, little details,
episodic events?

d. Is information
retrieved by recog-
nition, free recall,
or cueing?

e. Is recall increased
with:

- difference in task
(recall as many
fruits as you can
vs. recall the ones
that are fruit from
the word list
presented)
- giving a reward as
incentive to recall
- giving a memory
strategy (chunking,
imagery) as help?

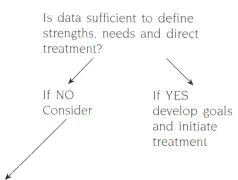

Is data sufficient to define strengths, needs and direct treatment?

If NO
Consider

If YES
develop goals
and initiate
treatment

SPEED OF INFORMATION PROCESSING

Is there evidence that slowed processing of information affects performance in communication?

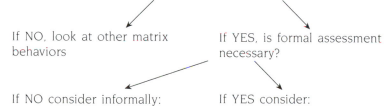

If NO, look at other matrix behaviors

If YES, is formal assessment necessary?

If NO consider informally:

1. Are responses based on visual input different from auditory?
2. If pauses are inserted when being given information, is response more accurate?
3. If response is not cued or question not repeated, how long does it take for response?
4. Is question forgotten if given too much time?
5. Are directions requested for same task frequently?

If YES consider:

1. Ross Information Processing Test (PRO-ED)
2. Formally time responses while giving information rapidly and with pauses

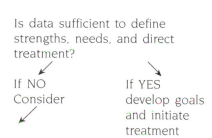

Is data sufficient to define strengths, needs, and direct treatment?

If NO
Consider

If YES
develop goals
and initiate
treatment

EXECUTIVE FUNCTIONING

Does behavior demonstrate possible problems with executive functioning that may affect performance in communication?

If NO, look at other matrix behaviors

If YES, is formal assessment necessary?

If NO consider informally:

1. What is cognitive understanding of personal strengths and needs?

2. Prior to formalized test how does child predict he/she will do?

3. How does child evaluate how he/she performed after subtest or test?

4. Can child set goals to achieve completion of a task (work or play) without external direction?

5. Is plan devised to attempt goals?

6. Is plan self initiated and appropriate to age?

7. Is problem solving skill used if a problem with the plan arises?

8. Do inappropriate behaviors interfere with completion of plan and does child try to inhibit these behaviors?

9. Is self talk employed to monitor behaviors during an activity?

10. Are there demonstrated abilities to evaluate self on completed test or therapy tasks?

If YES consider:

1. Ask for written or verbal analysis of perceived strengths and needs.

2. HAPI (age 15 and up)

3. Concept Formation subtest: Woodcock-Johnson (Psychoeducational Test Battery (DLM Teaching Resources)

4. Likeness/Differences subtest: DTLA-2 (PRO-ED)

5. Associations subtest: Word Test (Lingui-Systems)

Is data sufficient to define strengths, needs, and direct treatment?

If NO Consider

If YES develop goals and initiate treatment

11. Organization

    a. Is there ability to describe steps in an activity like baking a cake?

    b. Is there ability to describe tools needed to complete activity like mowing the lawn?

    c. Is there ability to sequence steps for activity like studying for a test?

    d. What ability to categorize (by class, function) is present?

    e. What ability to associate within, across, categories is noted?

RECEPTIVE LANGUAGE

Does understanding verbal or written communications suggest performance in communication may be affected due to receptive language problems?

If NO, look at other matrix behaviors

If YES, is formal assessment necessary?

If NO consider informally:

1. Is vocabulary at age level?

2. Does vocabulary development keep up after injury?

3. Are there gaps in curriculum specific vocabulary?

4. Is there a difference in ability to follow written vs. verbal directions?

5. Is there a difference in following directions if gestural or tactile information is provided?

If YES consider:

1. PPVT (American Guidance Service)

2. Woodcock-Johnson Psycho-Educational Test Battery (DLM)

3. Token Test for Children (DLM Teaching Resources)

4. Directions subtests, CELF (The Psychological Corporation)

5. Spelling and vocabulary tests from previous and present grade levels

6. Does rate, amount or complexity of information presented verbally or written affect receptive abilities?

7. Is there a difference in ability to comprehend based on communication demands of person, environment?

6. PIAT (American Guidance Service)

7. Test of Auditory Comprehension of Language: TACL-R (DLM Teaching Resources)

8. Refer to reading teacher for testing

Is data sufficient to define strengths, needs, and direct treatment?

If NO
Consider

If YES
develop goals
and initiate
treatment

EXPRESSIVE LANGUAGE

Do verbal or written communications suggest performance in communication may be affected due to expressive language problems?

If NO, look at other matrix behaviors

If YES, is formal assessment necessary?

If NO consider informally:

1. Are there oral-motor weaknesses (dysarthria, apraxia) noted?

2. Is there a problem swallowing various textures of food?

3. What is ability to use words in naming tasks related to familiar or unfamiliar context?

4. Is there a difference in verbal versus written output? (Using a detailed picture, if story is told, then written, what changes in ideas, word choice, details, grammar, occur?)

If YES consider:

1. Comprehensive Apraxia Test (Praxis House Publishers) Dysarthria Test

2. Frenchay Dysarthria Assessment (College-Hill Press)

3. Formal Dysphagia Assessment

4. Test of Word Finding (DLM Teaching Resources)

5. Word Association: CELF-R (The Psychological Corporation)

6. Rapid Automated Naming Test (Denckla & Rudel, 1974)

7. TOLD (PRO-ED)

5. What differences are noted in verbal output when topic of conversation is structured vs. unstructured?

6. When asked a question, is response tangential or on topic?

7. Is confabulation present and can it be redirected?

8. What is amount of verbalization? Is being withdrawn or hyperverbal in a conversation a concern?

9. Can information from several sentences be condensed into main idea (telegram)?

8. TOWL (PRO-ED)

9. The Word Test (Lingui-Systems)

10. The Adolescent Word Test (Lingui-Systems)

Is data sufficient to define strengths, needs, and direct treatment?

If NO
Consider

If YES
develop goals
and initiate
treatment

PRAGMATIC LANGUAGE

Do pragmatic language skills indicate potential difficulty in communication?

If NO, look at other matrix behaviors

If YES, is formal assessment necessary?

If NO consider informally:

1. Is disinhibition observed in conversation?

2. Is there a problem understanding use of social space (proxemics)?

3. Are non-verbals used appropriately?

4. Are non-verbals understood and responded to adequately?

5. In unstructured conversation:
   • what is ability to introduce topic?

If YES consider:

1. Pragmatic Protocol (Prutting & Kirschner)

2. Ross Test of Higher Cognitive Functions (Academic Therapy Publications)

3. Review expressive segments of language tests

4. The Adolescent Test of Problem Solving (TOPS) (Lingui-System)

5. Complete analysis of language sample

- what is ability to maintain topic?
- what are turn taking skills?
- what are turn giving skills?
- what are repair/revision strategies?
- what are specificity/accuracy skills?

Is data sufficient to define strengths, needs, and direct treatment?

If NO
Consider

If YES
develop goals and initiate treatment

None of these domains should be regarded in isolation; each has an impact on the other. By considering all aspects, the best idea about the potential of the child/adolescent with TBI to communicate within a given situation is obtained. A proactive approach to assessment of the child/adolescent allows descriptions of potential problems to be developed, and workable solutions proposed. These solutions are the focus of Part III of this text.

Summary Guidelines

1. Assessment must take multiple aspects into consideration to provide appropriate placement and intervention. We have more tools than a hammer and children with TBI are unique in their impairments and cannot all be considered nails!

2. There should be a combination of formal assessment and informal evaluation that provides a portfolio of information about the cognitive-communicative strengths and needs of the child/adolescent.

3. Functionally based evaluation and description provides much needed information that allows for the most integrated transitions to home, school, work, and community life.

4. Families should be involved participants in assessment.

5. Various processes of language—expressive, receptive, and pragmatic, as well as memory, perception, information processing, executive functioning, and attention—are interrelated and essential to defining the language strengths and needs of a child/adolescent with TBI.

6. Language is critical to the learning process.

7. Assessment is ongoing during the developmental years of the child/adolescent with TBI.

8. Transition from class to class, grade to grade, home to school, school to work is based on continued assessment of strengths and needs. These needs will be ever-changing.

References

Adamovich, B., & Henderson, J. (1992). *Scales of cognitive ability for traumatic brain injury.* Chicago: The Riverside Publishing Co.

Adamovich, B., Henderson, J., & Auerbach, S. (1985). *Cognitive rehabilitation of closed head injured patients.* San Diego: College-Hill Press.

Baxter, R., Cohen, S., & Ylvisaker, M. (1985). Comprehensive cognitive assessment. In Ylvisaker, M. (Ed.), *Head injury rehabilitation: Children and adolescents* (pp. 247–286). Boston, MA: Little, Brown and Co.

Begali, V. (1987). *Head injury in children and adolescents: A resource and review for school and allied professionals.* Brandon, VT: Clinical Psychology Publishers.

Blackwood, R. (1971). *Operant control of behavior: Elimination of misbehavior and motivation of children.* Akron, Oh: Exordium Press.

Blosser, J. L., & DePompei, R. (1992). A proactive model for treating communication disorders in children and adolescents with traumatic brain injury. *Clinics in Communicative Disorders, 2*(2), 52–65.

Carr, E. G., & Durand, V.M. (1985). Reducing behavior problems through functional communication training. *Journal of Applied Behavior Analysis, 18,* 111–126.

Cohen, S. (1991). Adapting educational programs for students with head injuries. *Journal of Head Trauma Rehabilitation, 6*(1), 56–63.

Cone, J. D. (1987). Behavioral assessment with children and adolescents. In M. Hersen & V. B. Van Hasslet (Eds.), *Behavior therapy with children and adolescents: A clinical approach* (pp. 57–71). New York: Wiley.

Day, R. M., Rea, J., Schlusser, N. G., Larson, S. G., & Johnson, W. L. (1988). A functionally based approach to the treatment of self injurious behavior. *Behavior modification, 12,* 565–589.

DePompei, R., & Blosser, J. L. (1987, April). *Facilitating classroom success for the closed head injured student.* Paper presented at Council for Exceptional Children, Chicago.

DePompei, R., & Blosser, J. L. (1991a). Families of children with traumatic brain injury as advocates in school reentry. *Neurorehabilitation, 1*(2), 29–37.

DePompei, R., & Blosser, J. L. (1991b). Functional cognitive-communicative impairments in children and adolescents: Assessment and intervention. In J. Kreutzer & P. Wehman (Eds.), *Cognitive rehabilitation for persons with traumatic brain injury: A functional approach.* Baltimore: Paul H. Brookes Publishing Co.

DePompei, R., & Blosser, J. L. (1993). Professional training and development for pediatric rehabilitation. In C. Durgin, N. Schmidt, & J. Freyer (Eds.), *Staff development and clinical intervention in brain injury rehabilitation* (pp. 229–253). Gaithersburg, MD: Aspen.

Donellan, A. M., Mirenda, P. L., Mesaros, R. A., & Fassberger, L. L. (1984). Analyzing the communicative functions of aberrant behavior. *Journal of The Association for Persons with Severe Handicaps, 9,* 201–212.

Duerk, B. (1990). Unpublished manuscript. University of Akron, Akron, OH.

Durand, V. M., & Carr, E. G. (1987). Social influences on self-stimulatory behavior: Analysis and treatment application. *Journal of Applied Behavioral Analysis, 20,* 119–132.

Durand, V. M., & Crimmins, D. B. (1988). Identifying the variables maintaining self-injurious behavior. *Journal of Autism and Developmental Disorders, 18,* 99–117.

Ewing-Cobbs, L., Fletcher, J., Levin, H., & Landry, S. (1985). Language disorders after pediatric head injury. In J. K. Darby (Ed.), *Speech and language evaluation in neurology: Childhood disorders* (pp. 97–112). Orlando, FL: Grune & Stratton.

Gerring, J. P., & Carney, J. M. (1992). *Head trauma: Strategies for educational reintegration.* San Diego: Singular Publishing Group.

Groher, M. E. (1990). Communication disorders in adults. In M. Rosenthal, E. Griffeth, M. Bond, & J. D. West (Eds.), *Rehabilitation of the adult and child with traumatic brain injury* (2nd ed.) (pp. 148–162). Philadelphia: F. A. Davis.

Harrington, D. (1990). Educational strategies. In Rosenthal, M., Griffeth, E., Bond, M., & Miller, J. D. (Eds.). *Rehabilitation of the adult and child with traumatic brain injury* (2nd ed.) (pp. 476–492). Philadelphia: F. A. Davis.

Kennedy, M. R., & Deruyter, F. (1991). Cognitive and language bases for communication disorders. In D. R. Beukelman & K. M. Yorkston (Eds.), *Communication disorders following traumatic brain injury: Management of cognitive, language, and motor impairments.* Austin, TX: PRO-ED.

Kreutzer, J. (1993). *Community reintegration: Assessment concerns.* Presentation at St John's Medical Center, Detroit, MI.

Kreutzer, J. S., & Wehman, P. H. (1991). *Cognitive rehabilitation for persons with traumatic brain injury.* Baltimore: Paul H. Brookes Publishing Co.

Lehr, E. (1990). *Psychological management of traumatic brain injuries in children and adolescents.* Rockville, MD: Aspen Publications.

Lennox, D. B., & Miltenberger, R. G. (1990). Conducting a functional assessment of problem behaviors in applied settings. *The Journal of the Association for Persons with Severe Handicaps, 14*(4), 304–311.

Milton, S., Scaglione, C., Flanagan, T., Cox, J. L., & Rudnick, D. (1991). Functional evaluation of adolescent students with traumatic brain injury. *Journal of Head Trauma Rehabilitation, 6*(2), 35–46.

O'Leary, K. D., & Wilson, G. T. (1986). *Behavior therapy: Application and outcome.* Englewood Cliffs, NJ: Prentice-Hall.

Rosen, C. D., & Gerring, J. P. (1986). *Head trauma: Educational reintegration.* San Diego: College-Hill Press.

Rosenthal, M., Griffeth, E., Bond, M., & Miller, J. D. (1990). *Rehabilitation of the adult and child with traumatic brain injury* (2nd ed.). Philadelphia: F. A. Davis.

Russell, N. (1993). Educational considerations in traumatic brain injury: The role of the speech-language pathologist. *Language, Speech, and Hearing Services in the Schools, 24*(2), 67–75.

Russell, N., & Grantham, R. (1992, April). *Traumatically brain-injured school children: Testing the limits/implementing compensations.* Paper presented at the New York State Speech-Language-Hearing Association, Kimesha.

Sohlberg, M. M., & Mateer, C. A. (1989). The assessment of cognitive-communicative functions in head injury. *Topics in Language Disorders, 9*(2), 15–33.

Telzrow, C. F. (1987). Management of academic and educational problems in head injury. *Journal of Learning Disabilities, 20,* 536–545.

Telzrow, C. (1991). The school psychologist's perspective on testing students with traumatic head injury. *Journal of Head Trauma Rehabilitation, 6*(2), 23–34.

Telzrow, C. F. (1994). Best practices in facilitating intervention adherence. In A. Thomas & J. Grimes (Eds.), *Best practices in school psychology* (3rd Ed.). Washington, DC: National Association of School Pyschologists.

Willams, J., & Kay, T. (Eds.). (1990). *Head injury: A family matter.* Baltimore: Paul H. Brookes Publishing Co.

Ylvisaker, M.(1985). *Head injury rehabilitation: Children and adolescents.* San Diego: College-Hill Press.

Ylvisaker, M. (1993). *Assessment and treatment of traumatic brain injury with school age children and adults.* Buffalo, NY: EDUCOM.

Ylvisaker, M., Chorazy, A., Cohen, S., Mastrill, J., Molitor, C., Nelson, J., Sezekeres, S., Valko, A., & Jaffe, K. (1990). Rehabilitative assessment following head injury in children. In M. Rosenthal, E. Griffeth, M. Bond, & J. D. Miller (Eds.), *Rehabilitation of the adult and child with traumatic brain injury* (2nd ed.) (pp. 558–584). Philadelphia: F. A. Davis.

Ylvisaker, M., & Goebbel, E. M. (1987). *Community re-entry for head injured adults.* Boston: Little, Brown.

Ylvisaker, M., & Sezekeres, S. (1994). Communication disorders associated with closed head injury. In R. Chapey (Ed.), *Language intervention strategies in adult aphasia* (3rd ed.) (pp. 546-568). Baltimore: Williams & Wilkens.

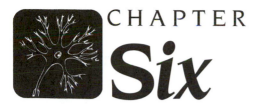

CHAPTER

Six

Scanning and Analyzing the Environment and People in the Environment

The success of service delivery for children with TBI depends not only on the services provided directly to the youngster but also on two additional elements: the environment in which the child must function and the people encountered within that environment. Assessment must consider not only the strengths and weaknesses of the child, but also the impact of these elements. It is important to identify demands and expectations the child will confront, obstacles that may interfere with or threaten success, and opportunities that will enable it. This information, combined with information obtained by assessing the child, provides the comprehensive data needed to develop workable treatment strategies. The goal of conducting an environmental analysis is to produce a data-based picture of the most significant environmental factors around which the program, goals, and objectives must be formulated.

Program planners should keep several questions in mind during assessments of the environment and people within the environment:

1. What are the cognitive-communicative demands of the situation?
2. What is the individual's capability to:
   - Attend to a task in order to complete it?
   - Attend with distractions present?
   - Shift attention from one activity to another?
   - Maintain the topic being discussed?
   - Maintain a conversation while working at another task?
   - Recall task sequence?
   - Follow oral and written instructions?
   - Ask for repetition when needed?
   - Use appropriate vocabulary?
   - Remember locations around work area?
   - Maintain appropriate social interactions?
3. What problems could arise because of the demands of the environment and the interactive communication characteristics of people in the environment?
4. What solutions to the problems can be proposed to aid in maintaining this individual within this environment?

Assessing the Environment: Searching for the Right Tools

The influence of environmental factors is frequently overlooked and not considered when planning reintegration and treatment programming for children with TBI. The nature of the environment in which a child lives, learns, plays, and works can contribute to successes and failures. Supportive environments can increase the potential for success in learning and interactions.

A number of environmental factors should be considered including: physical aspects, psychological climate, materials used, and social context.

It is easy to understand the influence of physical environmental factors if one considers their own personal reaction to features of their environment (such as temperature, noise, visual, and auditory distractions) when trying to concentrate on an important conversation or listen to difficult material. A child's location in a room might affect ability to attend to tasks and fully participate. For children with physical disabilities, physical barriers may result in decreased participation. The planning team must assess the accessibility of the facilities the child will enter, transportation needs, and basic needs such as feeding and toileting.

For each of these physically related situations, the environment will need to be prepared. In addition, the child will need to develop skills for participation, despite obstacles. This might mean incorporating assistance of equipment or people and/or strengthening the child's abilities to express needs and request help when needed.

A positive and supportive psychological climate results in higher performance. The level of enthusiasm and acceptance of the child displayed by others in a situation will provide needed encouragement. Other psychological aspects also can set the scene for facilitating skill development and improved performance, including patience, cooperativeness, active engagement, and motivational techniques (reinforcement, rewards etc.).

There are two ways to face the experience . . . sit down, feel helpless, sorry for myself, do nothing . . . or give it all I have with positive thinking, we-can-do-it attitude, and utilize the energies of many to help me conquer what seemed to be an impossible task. I told myself that every day I would have at least one positive objective in mind to get my child to where he needed to go. (Jason's Mom)

The materials a child interacts with can stimulate increased interest and better responses. Materials need to be selected with the child's developmental level and skill level in mind. Materials should be adapted according to specific needs. For instance, assistive devices, computers, and augmentative equipment should be available, if required. Graphic and pictorial symbols should be added to increase usability, if needed.

Perhaps the most important aspect of the environment is the social context. The interactions a child can be expected to have with other people should be evaluated, as well as the degree of structure and informality, plus the scheduling routine. What level of involvement with others will be required? What are the formats for participation? What rules guide activities and participation? What supports are needed from others to facilitate maximum inclusion and participation?

Environmental factors such as these can be evaluated formally through structured observations or informally via discussions and interviews with key people in the youngster's life. Once identified, an important part of taking a proactive treatment approach is manipulation of environmental factors such as these to benefit the child.

Demands and Expectations: Blueprints for Participation

Each situation in which a youngster participates carries with it numerous routines, demands, and performance expectations. It is often most difficult to determine a child's "readiness" for entering a given situation. As a beginning point, a description can be created of the type and level of skills needed for participation in a particular activity or situation. To illustrate this point, Table 6–1 provides a list of skills needed for successful participation in school and work situations. First, the evaluator determines the skill needed for success in the particular situation through interview and observational techniques. Next, clinicians, teachers, and family members who have worked with the youngster provide their assessment of the child's current level of performance in these skill areas. This provides family and others with a realistic description of expectations for the environment the child is being reintegrated into. It provides planners with concrete data for goal setting. Finally, it provides a method for assessing progress over time.

Table 6–2 lists some common requirements and expectations for children's interactive communication skills in home, school, and community situations. The child's capability for meeting each of these expectations needs to be determined. If capability is doubted because of the child's problems, expectations should be discussed and revised and strategies for developing the child's skills and providing support should be determined.

A reintegration into the school setting can serve as a good example of how to conduct an environmental assessment for that environment. Close contact should be kept with teachers before a youngster joins a teacher's class and throughout placement in the class. Educators should be interviewed to determine the cognitive/communicative requirements for success within the classroom setting and the student's present performance on educational and social tasks within that setting. Conducting an extensive evaluation of the classroom and teaching strategies employed (and the child's performance within the classroom when appropriate) yields valuable information for formulating an ongoing diagnosis and developing relevant intervention plans.

Many sources can be used to obtain valuable information about a child's performance and capabilities, including questionnaires, checklists, work samples, observations, compilation of data from others, and structured testing. Regardless of the evaluation format used, evaluation of the student's learning and social performance within specific environments should be ongoing. This is an important proactive problem-solving step, especially for reintegration into the school setting. Evaluation can be interwoven into all learning and interaction activities if those who work with the child learn to be astute observers and understand how to implement instructional and cognitive/communication interaction strategies in response to the behaviors they observe.

Table 6–1. Skills Needed for Transition Success

During the transition planning process:

I. Indicate the specific situation in which the youngster is expected to participate (class, family activity, community activity, or work task).

II. Identify skills needed or expected for successful participation in the particular situation.

III. Identify areas of strength or need presented by the individual. Indicate strengths with a plus (+) and needs with a minus (–). Summarize your findings by describing the individual's characteristic performance patterns at this point in time. Use your description during the planning process either prior to reintegration, after a period of reintegration, or for evaluating progress over time. In your description, specify those areas that will promote success and those that will inhibit it.

IV. Discuss findings at a planning meeting attended by the individual (if appropriate), family members, and significant professionals.

V. Formulate goals for treatment based on the findings.

Date of observation: _____ Observer: _____

Name: _____

Situation/s observed and targeted for transition: _____

Skills Needed for Successful Transition	Strengths	Needs Improvement	Target for Treatment; Planned Course of Action
Active learning • Participates in learning tasks • Takes initiative • Demonstrates motivation			
Awareness • Recognizes critical information • Responds to directions			
Communication efficiency • Oral and written communication skills enable learning and interactions			
Attention and concentration • Tunes in and stays on task			

(continues)

Table 6–1. (continued)

Skills Needed for Successful Transition	Strengths	Needs Improvement	Target for Treatment; Planned Course of Action
Information processing • Processes incoming information when presented at average speeds and amounts			
Self control • Inhibits impulsive and inappropriate behaviors • Accepts responsibility for decisions and actions • Works in spite of distractions			
Interactive learning • Engages in meaningful dialogue and interaction with communication partners • Gains information from books, learning, discussions • Asks and answers questions • Contributes to discussions			
Persistence • Stays on task until completed • Completes assignments			
Problem solving • Identifies problem situations, poses solutions • Generalizes information from one situation to another • Thinks about performance • Evaluates situations			
Organization • Follows established routines • Organizes materials and self for optimal learning • Moves from one activity to the next smoothly			
Recall • Displays accurate memory for info • Follows directions accurately			

***Table* 6-2.** Cognitive/communicative behaviors important for successful transition: Demands and expectations

Following are abilities in cognitive/communication behaviors that can affect the individual's ability to perform and communicate effectively with family, friends, and within school, community, and work.

Demands and Expectations Posed by Family-Related Situations

- Following family rules
- Responding to questions
- Participating in conversations in a give and take manner
- Respecting others
- Showing interest in family activities (baseball, chess, running, Scouts, poetry, music and so on)
- Expressing or withholding expression of feelings
- Completing household chores
- Comprehending written notes about who is where or what is to be done at home
- Controlling behavioral outbursts

School- and Work-Related Demands and Expectations

- Using appropriate phonology, syntax, semantics, and pragmatics to meet verbal and written expression requirements
- Responding appropriately when asked a question
- Understanding the meaning of vocabulary and concepts unique to subject areas
- Interacting socially
- Formulating and asking questions to obtain information
- Following written and spoken instructions
- Organizing thoughts
- Understanding word relationships

Friends and Community Demands and Expectations

- Using age-appropriate vocabulary (including slang expressions)
- Responding within adequate time (processing time is not so delayed as to "turn off" peers)
- Understanding puns, humor, sarcasm
- Participating equally in a conversation rather than monopolizing it
- Controlling anger and frustration
- Using "social space" appropriately (not standing too close or too far away)
- Controlling disinhibited speaking out
- Following the rules of a game or activity correctly
- Generalizing from one social situation to the next
- Formulating questions to obtain necessary information

Evaluations should focus on the student as a learner, communicator, and interactor. If significant changes are observed in the child's performance from one situation or context to the next, the reasons for the changes should be determined. They may be related to the physical environment, the manner and style of communication of the persons the child is with, or the child's ability to perform the task. Decisions regarding steps to take to help the child will be dependent on the cause of the problem.

Assessing People in the Communication Environment: Different Tools for Different Projects

In addition to assessing the individual and the environment, a third important step in the data gathering process is to obtain pertinent information about the persons with whom the individual will interact most frequently. This includes identifying who the communicators are and determining what they know (or must find out) about TBI and what to do to help those persons. It is most essential, however, to describe the interactive communication manner and style that key people in the child's life use and to determine the impact of their interactions on the child. Do their interactions serve to facilitate the best performance from the child or do they lead to misunderstandings, frustrations, and problems?

It is a widely accepted social phenomenon that one person's behavior can and does often influence another's. We have all observed situations in which one person in a conversation lowers the voice and others automatically do, too. We have also seen people lose their "train of thought" when distractions or noises are introduced during a discussion. We have had our thoughts re-directed after someone draws us back to a conversation by speaking our name. We have seen young children ask a question repeatedly and become frustrated because no one appears to be listening or answering them. These simple observations help us understand that one person's communicative behaviors can influence another's. Given this, it is easy to understand that a child's performance might be affected by the way a communication partner responds or by the tone of voice used in asking a question. Most people do not recognize that subtle situations such as these have occurred. More importantly, they don't realize the effect they have on a child's performance.

It is possible to isolate and identify the individual nuances exhibited by a key communication partner. Further, it is an effective treatment strategy to describe the effect of those nuances on the child's performance given the child's communicative strengths and needs as a result of the TBI. To implement this process, others must be taught to recognize their own interactive communication characteristics and manipulate their own behavior in order to gain improvement in the child's behavior. A process of identification and matching is used for identifying communication behaviors and matching them to the child's strengths and needs based on whether they will help or hinder the child.

There are many procedures professionals can use to obtain information about the communication characteristics of others. Table 6–3, "The Communication Style Identification Checklist" (Blosser, 1990; Neidecker & Blosser, 1993) presents a systematic method for helping people analyze and describe their own interactive communication manner and style. It can be used by a professional as a format for discussion in order to jointly assess the communication style and manner of a child's communication partners. Or, it can be given to them to be used independently as a self-evaluation tool.

Solicit the Youngster's Opinions About Needed Changes: All the Nails Are Different

Often one of the most ignored individuals in the treatment planning process is the person with the problem. Yet, we often find that seeking a youngster's insights and opinions about personal needs yields the most appropriate strategies for intervention. Clinicians can obtain good insights by asking several pertinent questions as demonstrated in the worksheet in Table 6–4. The worksheet is designed to be used as an interview guide or for the child to complete independently depending on the child's capabilities.

A Format for Focusing Discussion

The chart presented in Table 6–5 is a mechanism for focusing discussion on identifying environmental demands and expectations, as well as interactive communication characteristics of others that confront a child. It further encourages planners to specify obstacles to success and opportunities for making modifications. Recommended strategies for providing assistance to a child will evolve from discussions about these topics.

Summary Guidelines

1. The environment and people in the environment play an important role in the success of service delivery. Treatment planners should keep this in mind in developing program plans.

Table 6–3. Communication style identification chart.

Instructions

During conversations and interactions with _____ , pay close attention to your own communication manner and style.

As completely as possible, describe the characteristics of your own communication manner and style in the categories listed below.

In consultation with a speech-language pathologist, determine those characteristics that can potentially pose difficulty for the student. Place a minus (–) next to them. Place a plus (+) beside those behaviors that can be used to promote the use of good communication skills.

Based on the findings, determine what changes you might make that would have a positive effect on the child's interactions with you in learning, working, or social situations.

Communication Manner and Style Characteristics	Description of Your Personal Characteristics	How Might Your Characteristics Affect the Individual? Indicate (+) or (−)
Average rate of speech?		
Typical length and complexity of your sentences?		
Use of sarcasm, humor, or puns?		
Word choice (simple, difficult, technical)		
Attentiveness to people during conversations		
Organization of conversations		
Use of hand and body gestures		
Use of objects to help make explanations		
Manner of responding to questions others ask you		
Manner of giving directions or instructions		
Patience while waiting for someone else to talk or answer		
Ability to understand communication efforts		

***Table* 6–4.** Solicit the youngster's opinion about needed changes.

Let Us Know How To Help You

You are the best judge of how other people can cause problems for you or help you do better. Answer these 10 questions and let's work together to think of some helpful solutions.

1. What problems are you experiencing in class (at home, at work)? Briefly describe the problems you are having since you returned to school (your home, work, etc.).

2. How do you usually act when you are experiencing problems or frustrations in class (at home, at work)? List some of the ways you behave when you are having problems.

3. What classroom (home or work) situation causes you the most problems?
   • Noise
   • Temperature
   • Pictures and wall decorations
   • Other people in the room
   • Other things

4. List several ways your teachers (family, classmates, co-workers) help you when you experience trouble in class (at home or work).

5. What do you think people should do to help you?

6. List several things your teachers (classmates, co-workers) do to frustrate you or cause you more problems.

7. What do you think people should **stop** doing when they are around you?

8. At what time of day do you do your best? Why do you feel this is your best time of day?
   • Early morning
   • Mid-morning
   • Around noon
   • Mid-afternoon
   • Early evening
   • Late evening

9. If you could choose 3 skills to improve, what would they be?

10. Tell 5 things that are great about you that you wish other people would know.

Table 6–5. Format for discussing environmental expectations and interactive communication characteristics of others: Planning modifications.

Current status and skill level; readiness for participation	
Environmental demands and expectations	
Interactive communication characteristics of key people in the situation	
Obstacles to success	
Opportunities for making modifications	
Recommended strategies	

2. Goal setting must consider needs for specific communication behaviors in numerous environments.

3. Physical aspects, the psychological climate, the materials used, and the social context influence performance and, therefore, should be assessed to determine changes that can be made to increase the individual's potential for success.

4. Each situation encountered poses demands and expectations for cognitive-communication skills. These can be identified so the youngster can better understand them and learn to accommodate to them.

5. Family members and significant others such as teachers or employers can learn many of the intervention techniques clinicians employ. Such carryover of stimulation may be one of the most significant interventions therapists can achieve in treatment.

6. Each person with whom a youngster interacts has a unique communication manner and style that may help or hinder the performance. By characterizing that manner and style, we can promote greater understanding of the relationship to the youngster's performance and changes that can be made to improve opportunities for success.

7. Often the individual with the TBI is not asked to provide information and opinions about which strategies or techniques help or cause problems. Asking the youngster for ideas leads to greater understanding and improved treatment.

References

Blosser, J. (1990, February). *Making speech-language therapy relevant to education*. Presentation presented at Luczerne Public Schools inservice meeting, Luczerne, PA.

Neidecker, E., & Blosser, J. (1993). *School programs in speech-language: Organization and management*. Englewood Cliffs, NJ: Prentice Hall.

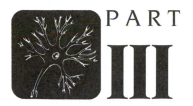

PART

III

Treatment of Cognitive-Communicative Strengths and Needs: An Interactive Approach

Merlin motioned "Come to the edge."
But they held back and said, "It is dangerous."
He beckoned, "Come to the edge."
And they said, "We may fail."
Then he commanded, "Come to the edge!"
So, they went to the edge and he pushed them. . . .
And they flew.

(Adapted from the words of Guillaume Apollinaire. Gordon, S., & Brecher, H. (1990). *Life is uncertain, eat dessert first*, p. 78. New York: Delacorte Press.)

Wouldn't it be wonderful if we could all be Merlin? To bring youth with TBI to the edge and make them fly is an art that many of us continue to develop. It takes a willingness to attempt new ideas, move into functional life situations with the child and include significant others in the process. Even then, we are still only learning to be "pushy" enough to help make them as effective in communication as we would like.

Just as with assessment, a proactive approach to treatment of cognitive-communicative impairments requires a perspective that subscribes to three interrelated aspects of communication:

A. Knowing the capabilities of the person with TBI and providing treatment to enhance strengths and rehabilitate or compensate for impairments;

B. Describing the demands of the environment and knowing what can be done to alter it;

C. Defining the capacity of persons in the environment to alter the demands for communication they impose on the child/adolescent, modify their communication mannerisms and behaviors via doable techniques to improve the child/adolescent's performance outcomes.

Cognitive-Communicative Performance Capabilities in Specific Situations

Cognitive-communicative impairments will interfere with performance in many situations. The impairments can be rehabilitated in some instances, compensated for in others, and must be accepted as incapable of being modified in still others. For example, the nonverbal child may be rehabilitated through motor strengthening and articulation exercises, may compensate with less than clearly articulated speech, or may have to abandon verbal speech as the primary means of communication and learn alternative communication with an augmentative device. Or a teacher who requires a student to answer questions verbally during discussion groups can allow one word responses or accept a different mode of response, such as pointing or writing.

Environmental Demands and Expectations for Communication

Following definition of a set of behaviors needed to perform successfully in a situation (including the characteristics, demands, and expectations of the environment), the environment can be altered to accommodate to the strengths or limitations of an individual. For example, the classroom in which many distractions are a problem can be altered with a study carrel or new seating arrangement.

It is also possible to determine that the environment cannot be modified or altered. For example, if the adolescent with TBI wants to attend a basketball game with friends, noise distractions in the gym will be present. Regardless of how distracting it is for that adolescent or how difficult it will be to concentrate on the game, as well as on social conversation and appropriate behaviors, the noise levels cannot be altered.

Communication Behaviors of Friends, Relatives, and Co-workers

Individuals in the communication environment can learn to alter or modify their responses and communication behaviors in many instances. In some situations, persons may be unable to alter behaviors to meet the needs of the child/adolescent with TBI. For example, a job coach may learn to slow the rate of speech when presenting new information to the adolescent with TBI. This same coach may not be able to change a vocal inflection pattern that the teen finds distracting and irritating. Figure III–1 is a model of this concept.

Our philosophy of treatment also requires that intervention be approached from a child-environment-centered perspective.

The Child-Environment-Centered Approach

Because learning is a primary task for children and adolescents and learning is a language-based process (Berlin, Blank, & Rose, 1980; Silliman, 1984; Wiig and Semel, 1980), success in transition and integration to home, school, and community is often dependent on the ability to communicate effectively. The child/adolescent with cognitive-communication problems will be at risk in any language/learning situation and treatment must reflect understanding of this dilemma.

The child/adolescent and the persons in the communication environment report parallel successes and disappointments in language/learning because there is an interactive relationship. If the child/adolescent's communication skills are to be altered, both the individual with TBI and the communication partner may need to modify behaviors. Treatment must be child-centered to increase strengths and to modify impairments. Child-centered treatment can focus on direct rehabilitation of cognitive-

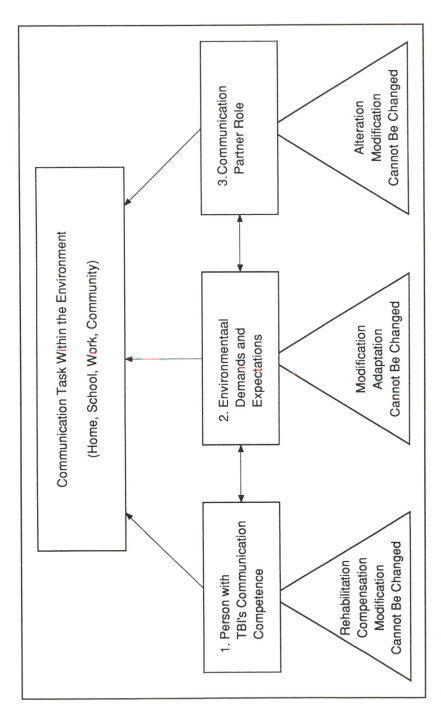

Figure III–1. Model for interactive intervention.

communicative impairments, teaching new compensatory communication behaviors and strategies, and one-on-one intervention based on positive reinforcement.

Treatment also must be environment-centered to provide communication partners the opportunity to modify both the environment and their own communication patterns. Environment-centered treatment focuses on the responsibilities of others to recognize that the person with TBI may be unable to alter all necessary communication behaviors. It implies that the environment itself or the persons in the environment hold equal responsibility for the communication success or failure.

Treatment, to be completely effective, must be both child and environment centered. It should be inclusive of all segments of the communication effort and various aspects of the treatment should often be inseparable. Treatment must be individualized and related to the functional needs of child/adolescent and the environment where performance or learning outcomes are expected. It must take into consideration transition and integration issues for the individual and recognize the complex interactions of these many factors. Treatment should be outcome based and rely on functional situations to determine success of the intervention. The chapters in Part III focus on suggestions for modification of the environment, ideas for outcome-based techniques for working directly with the child/adolescent, and methods for helping communication partners evaluate and alter their communication behaviors.

Readers should be able to:

1. Describe a child environment-centered approach to treatment that emphasizes the inseparable aspects of rehabilitation, transition, and continued success within home, school, community, and work.

2. Define general considerations for implementing treatment for the child/adolescent with cognitive-communicative problems.

3. Outline outcome-based treatment plans that include rehabilitation, compensation, and modification of behaviors, for the child/adolescent with TBI.

4. Understand procedures to modify or adapt the communication environment demands and expectations.

5. Suggest methods for helping communication partners understand responsibilities in communication situations and how to alter these behaviors.

References

Berlin, L. J., Blank, M., & Rose, S. A. (1980). The language of instruction: The hidden complexities. *Topics in Language Disorders, 1*(1), 47–58.

Silliman, E. R. (1984). Interactional competencies in the instructional context: The role of teaching discourse in learning. In G. P. Wallach & K. G. Butler (Eds.), *Language learning disabilities in school age children* (pp. 288–317). Baltimore: Williams and Wilkins.

Wiig, E. H., & Semel, E. M. (1980). *Language assessment and intervention for the learning disabled.* Columbus, OH: Charles E. Merrill.

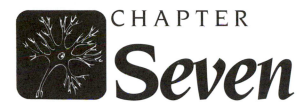

CHAPTER

Seven

Making Communication Work for the Child/Adolescent

Determining the most appropriate treatment for a child or adolescent with cognitive-communicative impairments following TBI is a complex process requiring considerable thought and planning. It is, therefore, important when determining treatment selection to understand the various aspects that can influence decision making about approaches and attitudes about treatment. This treatment section is based on the wealth of information provided by the following authors regarding proactive and innovative treatment for children/adolescents with TBI: Begali (1987), Beukelman and Yorkston (1991), Blosser and DePompei (1989, 1992), Cohen (1986, 1991), DePompei and Blosser (1991, 1993), Kreutzer and Wehman (1991), Milton (1988); Milton, Scaglione, Flanagan, Cox, and Rudnick (1991), Russell (1993), Sohlberg and Mateer (1989), Telzrow (1987, 1994), and Ylvisaker (1985, 1993). The chapter discusses general considerations for overall treatment planning and specific suggestions for intervention, including motor speech disorders, augmentative communication considerations, and receptive, expressive and pragmatic language interventions. Examples of functional goals, activities, and materials that can be employed to meet the goals and functional outcome criteria are outlined for each segment.

It's Time to Plan Treatment: General Concerns

A number of general concerns regarding treatment should be considered when planning goals and selecting treatment strategies.

Developmental Issues

Treatment should be planned with the age and developmental abilities of the individual in mind. Occasionally, professionals read suggestions for treatment that seem like excellent ideas, only to find the approaches unsuccessful when implemented. When analyzing what went wrong, often there will have been lack of consideration of the appropriateness of the level of material or the behavior expected because of a child's age or developmental readiness.

Preschoolers should have outcome goals for language and social experiences that reflect capabilities of most children in that age range. For example, preschoolers may be engaged in games such as pat-a-cake or play with dolls or trucks to stimulate appropriate level language experiences, with elementary-aged children more likely to benefit from games such as duck, duck, goose, hide-and-seek; concentration; or tic-tac-toe to involve appropriate developmental abilities. Adolescents should have goals that reflect problem-solving or executive-functioning skill development at higher levels. Deaton (1991) suggests they may be challenged by games such as Battleship (Milton Bradley), Connect Four (Milton Bradley), and poker or discussion about dating etiquette and relationships.

Materials and activities should be carefully examined for expected ability levels of the activity in relationship to the communication abilities of the individual for whom goals are being established. Expected outcomes for each activity also should reflect age or developmental levels appropriate for successful performance by each child/adolescent.

Socialization Issues

Children and adolescents use language as a means for development of socialization skills. Children and adolescents with TBI who have previously participated in daily life activities may find themselves limited in daily social interactions after the injury. Gillette (1994) suggests that this limited participation contributes to overall developmental delays, which include communication. She indicates that frequent and repeated experiences with both familiar and novel routines can contribute to a strong foundation for a wide variety of social and developmental issues, including communication. She recommends therapy for children focus on social routines that:

A. Keep a child with others in play and daily living routines;

B. Encourage a child to contact others to initiate a variety of routines

C. Challenge a child to converse for a variety of reasons and needs.

Goals and activities should reflect understanding of the need to maintain involvement in functional daily communication routines that encourage development of social communication skills.

Process Versus Strategy Training Issues

The retraining of such process-specific abilities as discrimination, memory, or attention has been discussed by authors such as Hagen (1988), Kennedy and Deruyter (1991), Parenté and Anderson (1983), Parenté and DiCesare (1991), and Sohlberg and Mateer (1989). Many retraining programs designed to provide training exercises for various processes are available commercially (*Brain Train* [Rehabilitation Psychology Associates, 1989]; *Captain's Log* [Sanford & Browne,1985]; *Cognitive Rehabilitation* [Smith, 1984]; *Attention Process Training* [Sohlberg & Mateer, 1987]; *Thinkable* [Psychological Corporation,1991]).

DePompei and Blosser (1991, 1993), Kreutzer (1993), and Ylvisaker (1993) suggest these process-specific interventions may not be as useful as once thought, because improvements in cognitive functioning do not seem to be demonstrated in carryover to activities of daily living. Ylvisaker (1993) indicates that there has been little research that demonstrates efficacy of process-specific intervention. He indicates that these decontextualized cognitive exercises have not demonstrated that abilities can be generalized to everyday tasks or that they are maintained over time. He also suggests that the exercises have no direct effect on communication effectiveness.

Treatment, if it is to be applicable to real-world situations, cannot begin and end with component training. Treatment directed toward increased attention, discrimination, sequencing, or memory without a specific behavior related to a functional task is not often so applicable. Communication skills, compensatory strategies, and functional performance in a given situation all play a part in personal-environment-centered treatment planning. Outcome-based strategy training, such as development of memory skills, language competencies, and executive functioning capacity related to functional behaviors needed to perform in a specific environment, is most relevant in making a difference in performance of daily activities. However, there is little evidence to demonstrate the effectiveness of this approach and there has been little research comparing process-versus-strategy training approaches. Therefore, therapists should look carefully at the benefits and weaknesses of all procedures and determine the best approach of treatment based on the needs of an individual child/adolescent.

Preschool, Elementary, Teenage Issues

As indicated previously, the age or developmental level of the child/adolescent should determine materials and approaches in treatment that are adequate and likely to be successful. It should be noted that certain areas might require attention depending on the age and developmental level demonstrated.

Preschoolers, regardless whether language delay is suspected, should receive intensive language stimulation through play and social situations. Parents should be taught to stimulate language and to watch for signs of emerging developmental delays.

Elementary children should receive stimulation for vocabulary development related to school work as well as social interchanges with friends and family. Introduction to simple memory strategies, problem-solving skills, and self-analysis of strengths and weaknesses are helpful.

Adolescents should concentrate on developing social interactions, maintaining ability to attend for longer periods of time, devising organizational skills for school and work, and determining realistic views of strengths and weaknesses in work, social, and school worlds.

Collaboration Issues

Children and adolescents with TBI will succeed only if many persons in their environment work collaboratively for successful intervention. One-on-one intervention in a quiet environment appears to be the least useful approach (except in early stages of recovery), as these children/adolescents must learn to cope with the stimulation and distractions of the real world. Therapy is most effective when jointly conducted by all important individuals in the child/adolescent's world. Communication takes place all day long with numerous individuals and treatment must involve those individuals. Therapists must be able to set transdisciplinary goals that can be accomplished with modeling, coaching, or education by all communication partners.

Functional Outcome-Based Goal Issues

If treatment is to be successful, it must be based in real-world activities. Cognitive-communication goals are easy to develop and relate to real-world situations, as communication forms the basis for most daily activity encounters. A preschooler should learn to participate in communication (play peek-a-boo, request desired items, follow simple family rules). Elementary-age children must learn to be a part of the daily routine at home (empty waste paper baskets, take turns at games, make shared TV choices), at school (follow directions, participate in classroom routines), and socially (turn take, use proper language with friends). A teen should learn to wait for rewards, participate in school learning and social routines, follow rules for work. All therapy activities should be directed toward the specific needs and abilities of a child/adolescent and goals should be developed based on environmental communication demands and the capabilities of the individual to meet those demands.

Strengths of the Child/Adolescent Issues

It is easy for therapists to focus on the impairments of the child/adolescent. However, there are always capabilities that remain after TBI. When assessment is completed, there should be several strengths that are apparent and these abilities should not be overlooked in the development of treatment plans. Rewards can be based on interests and abilities. Remediation of cognitive-communicative weakness can be built on areas of competence or interest.

Areas of strength should be documented in written reports and presented verbally to the child/adolescent and family. By recognizing and utilizing strengths, persons with TBI can be motivated to work and learn. Families can find encouragement to face weaknesses by knowing that some strengths are present. Self-esteem of the individual and family can be strengthened. Therapists may find pleasure in delivering information about strengths and may develop a different view of their client and family as well!

Rehabilitation, Modification, and Compensation Issues

Some skills of a child/adolescent can developed over time. Others can be stimulated through rehabilitation. Most can be modified to meet challenges in the environment. Many can be developed as compensations, which implies a conscious effort to employ a strategy or aid as a means to complete a task. It is also possible that a few cannot be altered because of the severity of an injury. Understanding of these concepts is central to the development of goals for treatment and essential to the selection of treatment materials.

Recognition that skill levels can be the goal of rehabilitation or objectives of compensation strategies selected also must guide decisions about when to initiate treatment and when to discontinue. There will be situations when children/adolescents simply need time to develop or when treatment is no longer indicated. Decisions must be based on a team's ability to determine when rehabilitation, modification, and compensation goals have been achieved or cannot be so. We must be willing to discontinue a process, preserve funds and time, allow others to try a different way, and reevaluate, if indicated. Treatment cannot go on for ever and many cognitive-communicative impairments cannot be restored to preinjury levels.

If thinking and planning are collaborative and transdisciplinary, there will always come a time when an individual and family are responsible for cognitive-communication and therapists are no longer needed. Reaching that time is the ultimate goal of therapy.

Shared Vision

Goals of therapy must be established and altered based on a shared vision of what is hoped for and what is possible. Professionals do not own the vision and should not attempt to direct therapy without input from the child/adolescent and family. Modification of goals may be dependent on the vision of the family rather than the vision of the therapist. By developing reasonable goals based on input from a variety of sources, the most realistic planning and modification can be developed and achieved.

Activity and Material Selection

There are a variety of activities and materials that are applicable to this population. Many are commercially available. Many can be created, based on the specific communication needs within a particular environment. Selection and application of activities and materials should be based on an individual's needs and not on availability of resources on the shelf or because of text or advertisement recommendations.

Stage of Recovery

Ylvisaker (1985, 1993) and Ylvisaker et al. (1990) outline early, middle, and late stages of recovery and suggest there are major emphasis changes in treatment, dependent on a child/adolescent's place in the various stages. Any planning for treatment must consider the overall cognitive and physical abilities of a child/adolescent and must account for additional changes expected during the movement from early to middle to late stages of treatment. For example, implementation of a comprehensive augmentative device for a child who may still recover verbal speech skills may be an unnecessary expenditure of therapist energy and financial resources; or planning to teach a teen to determine the main ideas in a lecture when there is little ability to maintain attention or vigilance to complete such a task, is not appropriate to the stage of recovery exhibited.

I have to keep thinking of what I can do for Jason to keep climbing up the mountain, because there is only one way and that is up! Even though I realized that the mountain was very steep, I couldn't look at it all at once. (Jason's Mom)

Let's Get Down to Business: Specific Cognitive-Communicative Interventions

Some aspects of treatment of the child/adolescent with TBI have been handled for years with other populations by speech/language pathologists. Most professionals have within their armamentarium a variety of techniques, activities, materials, and treatment procedures that will be successful with this population. Traditional treatment approaches to motor problems, anomia, vocabulary development, memory compensation, receptive and expressive language development, and so on can and should be incorporated into planning. However, the key to reasonable planning continues to be making therapy relevant to a person's unique environment and to outcome-based goals for that environment.

Individual-outcome-based goals for various environments should encompass skill development in a variety of communicative situations. To be effective, treatment needs to be functionally based and focus on development of four major outcomes:

- Participation in the learning process,
- Development of skills that make a person employable,
- Understanding of social skills needed for communication at home, school and work, and
- Development of independent living skills.

To promote program coordination between disciplines and among all team members, these four outcomes should be used as a framework for planning interventions. Table 7–1 illustrates the types of skills that can be targeted within each of the four main outcome areas.

Children/adolescents with cognitive-communicative impairments may have a variety of competency levels that need attention. Often some individual work is necessary to prepare a youngster to participate in real-world situations. Following is a series of suggestions for individualized

Table 7–1. Individual skills necessary for effective communication in various environments.

School	Employment
maintain adequate vocabulary	attend regularly
request information	communicate effectively
respond to questions	follow directions
follow directions	organize day and job routines
comprehend lectures	adapt to changes
read for functional comprehension	recognize mistakes
write for functional expression	correct mistakes
organize for planning and sequencing	care for work area
store and recall information for later use	ask for help
learn alternative study skill strategies	use appropriate manners
	use appropriate language
	demonstrate initiative
	cope with constructive criticism
Social	**Independent Living**
monitor actions	plan daily routine
manage time	carry out daily routine
understand cultural diversity	use public transportation
respect others	know community resources and how to access
use correct pragmatics	advocate for self without offending others
	manage finances

treatments, intended as a general series of suggestions or examples not geared to any age or severity level. Suggestions for intervention and materials are not finite and many other sources and procedures can be used successfully. Each example provides a single goal and outcome as a suggested model of what can be developed based on environmental expectations and needs. Modifications are always necessary, depending on unique circumstances of a particular child/adolescent. Materials suggested and publishers are listed in Appendix C.

When one of a mother's children is wounded, imagination and creativity have no boundaries! One of the therapists came into the room and saw all of the items I had purchased to help Jason and she asked if I was a therapist. I chuckled to myself and said "I'm just the mom." (Jason's mom)

Motor Speech Disorders

Motor speech disorders can result from TBI when injury disrupts the planning or execution of movements for speech production. Problems can include apraxia, dysarthria, phonation, respiration, and articulation disorders. Severity can be mild to severe. Therapists have long treated these types of impairments in children/adolescents as a result of other neurological disorders. When motor speech disorders are a problem for the child/adolescent with TBI, traditional approaches to remediation are usually helpful. These approaches, depending on personal orientation, might include oral motor exercises, thermal stimulation, and rehabilitation and compensation for phonation, respiration, articulation, and resonation problems.

Special Considerations

- Cognitive levels of the child/adolescent need to be understood, so that attention, direction following, or initiation or suppression of responses are compensated for during therapy.

- Apraxia implies motor initiation and planning disabilities. The nature of TBI may confuse the diagnosis of apraxia because cognitive involvement may cause a child/adolescent to appear to have apraxia when the impairment is of higher level executive functioning and planning processes. Careful assessment and intervention based on the implications of problems with higher level functioning versus a true apraxia is necessary.

- Stimulation of olfactory or tactile senses may facilitate oral motor movements.

- Rehearsal of isolated phonemes or CVC sets that are not real words may not stimulate recall of language previously learned and may not be relevant to a child/adolescent. Moving from oral motor exercises to phonation and immediately to meaningful words may be the most useful procedure.

- Unrelated word lists for speech production exercises may not be useful. When working with a phonological process, rather than using traditional word lists for a series of phonemes, it may be more useful to develop vocabulary from class spelling lists, science class vocabularies, social or work situations that can be practiced and used in the immediate environment with family and friends.

Functional Outcome Based Plan

I. School

    A. Goal: To teach compensatory articulatory movements for science and health vocabulary words to be spoken verbally in class.

        1. Activities:

            a. Oral motor exercises for tongue, lips, and jaw.

            b. Phonation exercises to increase intensity of voice production.

            c. Review of articulatory movements for sound production of various phonemes.

            d. Modeling, tactile and auditory stimulation for production of vocabulary words.

        2. Materials:

            a. Mirrors, tongue blades, Visi-pitch (instrument for pitch display), graphs, and pictures.

            b. Vocabulary word lists obtained from classroom teacher. If a child/adolescent is not in school, obtain previous vocabulary lists from the school.

            c. Treatment section of developmental apraxia of speech chapter in *Treating Disordered Speech Motor Control for Clinicians by Clinicians* (Marquardt & Sussman, 1991).

            d. Motor speech disorders chapter (Yorkston & Beukelman, 1991) in *Communication Disorders Following Traumatic Brain Injury*.

    B. Outcome criteria: Child will produce 65% of vocabulary words that are intelligible to persons other than the therapist. Production will occur in a structured environment (person asks for word) 80% of the time and in spontaneous speech (as word is called for in conversational speech) 65% of the time.

II. Employment

    A. Goal: To increase teen's intelligibility when requesting information about a job task.

        1. Activities:

            a. Oral exercises to strengthen tongue and lip movements.

            b. Breath control exercises to increase amount of phonation per exhalation.

            c. Practice on production of words needed within job task (pins, push, place, turn, enter, box, computer, numbers etc.).

            d. Rehearse formulation of questions related to job task.

            e. Practice verbal production of questions related to job task.

            f. Develop alternative method of asking questions if verbal production is unintelligible.

2. Materials:
   a. Oral motor exercises such as those found in Kilpatrick (1976) or Kilpatrick and DePompei (1986).
   b. Oral motor stimulation exercises presented in *Innovative Concepts: Speech and Language Newsletters,* (Rosenwinkel-Marsalla, 1983–1989).
   c. Vocabulary from job obtained from job coach or work supervisor. If teen has not returned to work, obtain old job vocabulary and use to stimulate language recall and prepare for possible return.
B. Outcome criteria: Teen will formulate questions about the job task and be understood 70% of the time. Alternative means of questioning will account for additional comprehension by the communication partner 20% of the time.

III. Social
A. Goal: To increase intelligibility so that good friends will understand single words and short sentences in conversational situations.
   1. Activities:
      a. Learn production of vocabulary related to interests of child and friends (Barney, T-Ball, Barbie, McDonalds meals, and so on)
      b. Practice production of one-word or short-phrase responses such as "right on" and "cool" that can help keep the child in the conversation.
      c. Teach alternative response modes, if necessary
   2. Materials:
      a. Vocabulary associated with interests and activities of friends.
      b. Materials commercially available in catalogues from Communication Skill Builders, Speech Bin, Midwest Publications.
   3. Commercial materials that develop social awareness such as *Towards Affective Development (TAD)* (American Guidance Service) or *Self-Esteem in the Classroom* (Self-Esteem Seminars)
B. Outcome criteria: Child will maintain intelligibility with selected vocabulary at 85% correct level with therapist and family. Child will be understood by friends in unstructured conversation about practiced vocabulary items at 75% level.

IV. Independent Living
A. Goal: To improve teenager's ability to be understood when requesting or giving information in public areas, such as a restaurant or drug store.
   1. Activities:
      a. Exercises to develop rate control.

    b. Breath control exercises for phrasing of sentences.

    c. Production exercises related to specific vocabulary for experience (ordering pizza over the phone, asking where shaving cream is located)

    d. Teach alternative means of requesting information if unable to be understood verbally.

  2. Materials:

    a. Rehearse production in real world situations such as conversations provided in Kilpatrick and DePompei (1986).

    b. Maintain a set of menus, newspapers with theater times, sports events, mall advertisements, mail coupons, phone books.

    c. Actually implement the rehearsed activity in real-world situations.

B. Outcome: Teenager will order pizza over the phone, order in a restaurant, ask for information in a drug store with 75% intelligibility. Teenager will compensate for misunderstood message by alternative means of communication 85% of the time.

Dysphagia

Some children/ adolescents will have difficulties with feeding and swallowing after a TBI. Whenever motor speech disorders are present or when the child/adolescent has chewing or swallowing difficulties, a dysphagia evaluation, including videofluoroscopic examination, must be completed and appropriate interventions initiated.

Special Considerations

There are a number of confounding factors, such as reduced cognitive abilities, inability to self-initiate or inhibit, difficulty with attention, lessened cognitive-communicative abilities, poor ability to follow directions, motor problems, severity of injury, developmental concerns, and relationship of the swallowing problem to other physical and perceptual impairments, that are significant factors for consideration in dysphagia evaluation. The interaction of all these factors must be understood when developing a safe feeding and swallowing intervention that meets the physical and cognitive needs of an individual.

    Dysphagia assessment and treatment is relatively new and requires significant training. It is unethical to initiate treatment for a child/adolescent without adequate training in this area. For this reason, no specific goals, interventions, or outcomes are outlined in this chapter. Each situation will be unique and planning should take cognitive-communicative status, physical competencies, modifications, and compensations possible into consideration. For information about dysphagia the reader is referred to the following authors: Bosma (1980, 1986, 1992), Groher (1992); Kaslon and Ruben (1978); Kenny, Kohiel, and Greenberg (1989); Klein (1981); Lazarus (1991); Langfitt and Gennarelli (1982); Lazarus and Logemann (1987); Logemann (1983); Mollitt, Golladay, and Seibert (1985); Morris and Klein (1987); Morris (1989); Patrick and Gcisel (1990); and Wilson (1977).

Dysphagia (Editor, R. Jones), contains numerous articles of importance for TBI. *The Journal of Head Trauma Rehabilitation* (Eds. Rosenthal & Berrol, 1989, 4,4) has also published an issue on dysphagia and traumatic brain injury. A tutorial in pediatric feeding/swallowing problems is published in Vol. *1*, No. 4. [Dec] *Journal of Medical Speech-Language Pathology* (Arvedson et.al.) Additionally, there are numerous seminars and workshops held throughout the country that can provide clinicians with helpful information and hands-on training for dysphagia. It is advised that no child/adolescent be evaluated or treated by a therapist who has not had additional seminar or course work and clinical experience with swallowing or feeding problems.

More milestones! Jason's speech therapist decided to try orange sherbet to see how his swallow reflexes would be. I told her that he would like chocolate ice cream better! (Jason's Mom)

Nonverbal/Augmentative Intervention

Little information is available about the numbers of children/adolescents who are nonverbal following TBI. Because of the nature of the injury, many are unable to speak during early stages of recovery. Depending on the severity of the cognitive-communicative impairments and the motor disabilities, some recover verbal skills quickly and a small number remain nonverbal for a lifetime. Planning and treatment of nonverbal skills is dependent on determining and understanding the stage of recovery, the severity of communication disorder, and the functional needs for communication at the time. Therapists need to have completed specialized training in the application and selection of assistive devices prior to working with this important aspect of communication. Considerations and materials for functional planning are based on the work of Beukelman and Mirenda, (1992); Deruyter and Kennedy, (1991) and Gillette (1993).

Special Considerations

- The needs for communication may vary with cognitive levels. A child/ adolescent in Rancho Los Amigos Medical Center Level of Cognitive Functioning III may only require help with developing a method of responding to simple questions or indicating functional needs, with an individual in higher function levels desiring to express wants, participate in information transfer, and be involved in social exchanges.

- Selection of augmentative systems, vocabulary, and treatment strategies is dependent on the different interactive needs of each cognitive level.

- Because there is alteration in behavior over time (some rapid change and some slowed or plateaued), the need for use of an augmentative device may diminish over time. Therefore, recommendation for extensive devices early in the recovery process may not be warranted.

- Deruyter and Kennedy (1991) report that the nonspeaking population of TBI have typically slower assessment and recovery processes, because the injuries are typically more severe.

- It is important to determine how the communication device will be used. Various needs include assessment, communication, rehabilitation, integration into home, school, community or a combination of uses. The interactive needs and the cognitive levels of a child/adolescent with TBI are critical in selection of equipment.

- It is important to avoid developing a device that allows a child/adolescent to communicate words or ideas that they are able to communicate in other ways. Motivation for learning to use a device that is too simple may be compromised by selection of a communication system that is not appropriate to the communication needs of the child/adolescent.

- There is not enough research data available to allow therapists to predict the likelihood of recovery of natural speech. Devices that supplement the communication process, regardless of the recovery stage, are considered necessary to healthy communication for a child/adolescent.

- Use of an augmentative device is not an either/or situation. Rather, use of augmentative communication (AC) should be considered a supplement to other means of communication.

- Although spelling may be a slow technique for some social language skills, it may be more effective if memory for symbols is a problem. Consider letter category coding, if speech is an issue and memory for new symbols is poor.

- Underlying cognitive-communicative processes must be considered when planning treatment with AC. The ability to attend, learn a new symbol system, and/or recall symbols when needed may severely impair the ability to adapt to a communication system. Even when a child learns a set of symbols, lack of carryover to functional use, due to memory problems over time, may interfere with adequate use of the system.

- Because of the combination of disabilities possible in TBI, multidisciplinary team evaluation is essential to determine all aspects of necessary treatment. Physical posturing, eye-hand movements, and potential for various methods of response (eye blink, hand movement, head nod) should be explored by professionals of various fields.

- The practicality of a communication system must be experienced by the child/adolescent, family and all other significant communicators in the environment for there to be a commitment to practice and use of the device.

Functional-Outcome-Based Plan

I. School:
  A. Goal: To develop cognitive skills of categorizing, sorting, discrimination for math (addition) using an augmentative system.
    1. Activities:
      a. Use communication board to develop category of objects and number of objects per category.
      b. Sort pictures by category and number.
      c. Use system for response to questions about how many are in a particular category.
      d. Try estimating number of beans and pennies in jar, flowers in patch, balloons or birds in sky by sorting or combining categories and responding with augmentative system.
    2. Materials:
      a. Pictures of categories desired.
      b. Math vocabulary word lists obtained from classroom teacher. If the child/adolescent is not in school, obtain previous vocabulary lists from the school.
      c. If dedicated funds for portable devices are not available, consider computer programs such as touch communication for *Power Pad*; talking touch window for *Touch Window*; or talking word programs such as *Key Talk*.
      d. Use *Features of Portable Communication Devices*, a two-poster wall chart of alternative augmentative communication (AAC) device characteristics (Kraat & Sitver-Kogut, 1993).
  B. Outcome criteria: Child will successfully use the augmentative device to sort or categorize sets in preparation for addition in math 90% correctly for the therapist and will respond in the classroom using the augmentative device 80% to teacher questioning.

II. Employment
  A. Goal: To improve teenager's ability to use an augmentative device interactively with employer to discuss needed adaptations of work station to fit physical needs.
    1. Activities:
      a. Determine needs of teenager to complete tasks on assigned job.
      b. Program the device for vocabulary needed on job.
      c. Practice on production of words needed to discuss adaptations of work station.
      d. Rehearse formulation of questions related to job task.
      e. Practice use of augmentative device in simulated conversation with employer.
    2. Materials:
      a. Devices from companies such as Adaptive Communication Systems, Cannon Corporation, Prentke Romich, Innocomp, Sentient Systems Technology, Words+ Inc., or Zygo Industries.
      b. Vocabulary for conversation programmed into device.
  B. Outcome criteria: Teenager will use augmentative device in interactive manner with employer to discuss adaptations needed for success on the job and employer will respond with understanding about requests and feasibility of those requests. Employer will report on ability to interactively discuss the concerns.

III. Social
  A. Goal: To increase family and hospital personnel's ability to use single pictures or objects to obtain yes-no responses for functional needs in the hospital by use of AC.
    1. Activities:
      a. Determine specific needs for communication, such as drink, food, TV, family members' names.
      b. Practice attending to familiar pictures, objects.
      c. Develop picture board with familiar objects, pictures.
      d. Determine method of responding by yes-no to questions about pictures or objects.
      e. Practice production of yes-no responses.
    2. Materials:
      a. Vocabulary lists obtained from staff and family.
      b. Custom developed personal pictures communication board.
      c. Consider use of commercially available picture systems such as packages from Imaginart Communication Products or Mayer-Johnson Co.
  B. Outcome criteria: Child will respond with 85% accurate yes-no responses to therapist, staff and family.

IV. Independent Living

    A. Goal: To increase teen's active involvement in transitional planning session with school, family, and vocational rehabilitation counselor to plan for move to vocational training through use of an augmentative system to communicate .

        1. Activities:

            a. Help teenager determine hopes for vocational training and program vocabulary into system.

            b. Practice interactive questioning and answering using augmentative system.

            c. Teach teenager the process for participating in a transition conference (who will be there, forms to be signed, reports that will be presented, etc.).

        2. Materials:

            a. Forms and charts found in Wehman (1992).

            b. Vocabulary necessary to be programmed into system.

            c. Information, charts found in Lash and Wolcott (in press)

    B. Outcome: Teenager will participate as active member in transition conference and will present opinions and requests that are understood by other participants 90% of the time. Verbal communication will be supplemented by the AAC device when necessary to achieve 90% criteria.

Language Intervention

Language problems in TBI can be mild to severe. Interventions should take into consideration the receptive abilities, expressive competencies, and pragmatic performance of a child/adolescent in various situations. Many of the traditional language stimulations and interventions will be useful with this population. Exercises to increase receptive language skills for recognizing vocabulary, following directions, and receiving information at varying rates, complexities, and amounts will provide additional competencies. Treatment for expressive language skills may include vocabulary development, formulation of questioning and answering techniques, expressions of self verbally and in writing, competence in conversational speech, and ability to provide verbal responses under varying demands (stress, rate, complexity, finding main idea, determining solutions) for those responses. Therapy to provide additional competence in pragmatic language skills includes teaching turn taking and requesting, topic maintenance, nonverbal responses, self-initiating and inhibiting, recognition and control of confabulations, tangential and hyperverbal speech. It may also include activities to develop executive functioning.

Special Considerations

- All cognitive-communicative processes are interrelated and "pure" language disability (aphasia) is rare in TBI. The interrelationship of all processes to language must be recognized and accounted for in language intervention.

- Anomia is described as a major characteristic of language problems within this population. In some cases, difficulties with higher cognitive functioning and memory create the appearance of anomia. When preparing plans for treatment, consideration of underlying processes of language and how these are affecting language performance is important.

- Tangential and hyperverbal speech may confuse family members and professionals about the need for language intervention. Careful analysis of verbal content and modification of output, as well as treatment of pragmatic language skills will often provide considerable improvement in the quality of the verbal communication.

- Drills of vocabulary words or sentence structure without application to a meaningful context are not usually helpful for the child/adolescent. Employing word and sentence usage for functional conversational development seems the most reasonable. Use of unrelated word lists, as opposed to vocabulary from work, school, family, social interests, does not seem beneficial.

- The actual situation is the best place to develop, compensate, or modify receptive and expressive skills. If participation with significant people (family, teacher, peers) or in an actual place (school, drug store, pizza parlor) is not possible, simulation of events can be helpful.

- It may be important to begin therapy in a quiet environment. However, moving to noisier, more realistic environments (cafeteria, back of classroom, physical therapy gym) may present a better picture of language competence in real-life situations.

- Controlling the environment by reducing distractions will often point out problems with memory process rather than weak attention skills.

- Milton (1988) suggests that therapists employ task analysis when developing treatment plans that can be applied to any number of functional daily situations. This approach to therapy—taking treatment to the environment where the individual will be required to perform and developing compensatory strategies based on the needs of the environment helps develop success in the environment. She outlines a method of defining the elements in the task, describing potential communication problems that may interfere with completion of the task, listing strengths that may assist with completion of the task, and devising compensatory strategies to assist with successful completion of the task. Table 7–2 is an example of this procedure.

Table 7–2. Task analysis example.

Task	Weaknesses	Strengths
Writing memos to immediate supervisor	May embed several thoughts into one sentence; Use of lengthy sentence construction made it difficult to extract individual thoughts May state main idea midway through a paragraph; Main idea became "buried" among preceding support sentences May use pronouns with an unclear or ambiguous referent May "beat around the bush" and be too general when attempting to convey specific thoughts May move abruptly onto new ideas or topics without providing smooth, integrative transitions between old and new content Overuse of sophisticated phraseology, which detracted from communicating thoughts effectively	Generally employed appropriate grammatical and word selection skills Able to recognize most errors or problems after the fact Willing to accept corrective feedback Recognizes the benefit of using strategies to perform task Able to apply identified strategies to subsequent situations Highly motivated to improve skill level

Compensatory Self-Evaluative Memo Writing Strategies

1. Mark where each sentence ends.
2. Evaluate the length of each sentence.
3. Evaluate how clearly each sentence conveys your thoughts. Ask yourself:
   (a) Am I using simple, short sentence structure?
   (b) Does this sentence read easily?
   If the answer is "no" for any of the above questions, then ask yourself:
   (a) 1-2-3. What am I basically trying to communicate in this sentence? (Be spontaneous when you answer this question. DO NOT focus on sentence sophistication. You can polish up your act later.)
   (b) How can I communicate my intent using several sentences?

(continues)

Table 7–2. (continued)

4. Reread memo and monitor for the flow of information. Guidelines include:
   (a) Establishing topic in the first sentence of each new idea. It generally works better to establish topic near the beginning of the sentence.
   (b) Evaluate integration among sentences. Ask yourself if the sentences are cohesive.
   (c) Evaluate each pronoun. Determine whether a clear referent is established. When in doubt, do not use the pronoun.

Source: Reprinted from Milton, S. (1988). Management of subtle cognitive communication deficits. *Journal of Head Trauma Rehabilitation,* 3(2), pp. 7&8, with permission of Aspen Publishers, Inc, © 1988.

It is imperative that a procedure such as task analysis be completed when designing treatment programs to remediate cognitive-communicative disorders.

• Organization abilities are essential to language treatment with this population. It is important to include experiences in developing ability to sort, classify, categorize, associate, and sequence in treatment planning.

• Social skill development requires self-analysis and awareness. Often for those with frontal lobe injuries, it is difficult to promote self-understanding about behaviors that are socially unacceptable. This segment of therapy sometimes becomes a battleground for therapist and child/adolescent, with the therapist insisting that the child "accept" deficits and stop "denying." The child/adolescent, who has recall of previous social skills attempts to have the therapist understand "how it was" and that to the youngster's way of thinking nothing is any different in post-TBI social interactions.

Several approaches are available for this problem area. Direct confrontation may work if potential for change (less frontal lobe involvement) is present. These include peer critiques, forced self-analysis by video review of behaviors or recitation of "report cards" from therapists and/or teachers. Use of these approaches is dependent on the child/adolescent's emotional balance, availability of support systems, and trust of the therapist.

Other less confrontational techniques may include use of log books, reviewing videos of behaviors with agreed on checklists to find appropriate behaviors as well as those which could have been done differently, allowing the child/adolescent to enter into an actual social activity and helping to determine later if it was successful or how it failed.

It is important that therapists recognize the futility of the argument regarding who is right or wrong about a behavior. "What if" problem-solving discussions may never be resolved as to what the correct approach might be. Or the child/adolescent will provide a correct response only to be unable to put the action into practice in the real-world, "what if" situation. Approaching social skill development through practical and functional activities and teaching self-analysis based on the results of task performance may be the most practical means to developing positive self-awareness within social contexts.

- Teaching adequate conversational skills based on commonly used terms, popular slang expressions, and topics of mutual interest may be helpful in keeping the child/adolescent in acceptable conversations with peers and family.

- Maintaining a file on age-appropriate comic strips, cartoons, jokes, and riddles helps establish sense of humor and ability to use language in more abstract ways.

- The use of popular tabletop games can be valuable tools for cognitive-communicative stimulation and retraining. Deaton (1991) suggests games have several advantages. They are inexpensive, readily available, rewarding and motivating, familiar to the child/adolescent, different each time played, enjoyable, and typically nonthreatening. She suggests multiple uses and applications for game use in a treatment program.

Functional Outcome-Based Plan: Receptive Language

I. School:
  A. Goal: To develop awareness of the amounts of auditory information that may be presented in the classroom and to provide means for adapting to the information presented or to compensating for information provided.
    1. Activities:
      a. Teach to listen for information: what is the main point, what are the central themes, ideas, what is the important vocabulary?
      b. Develop ability to self analyze attention skills for class: what is ability to block visual or auditory distractions; how long can attention be held?
      c. Develop ability to request additional or missed information.
      d. Develop recognition that some persons speak too rapidly and how to request repetition or slowing of rate.
      e. Read paragraphs of varying length to the child/adolescent and ask for recall (immediate and over periods of time).

Teach how to listen for important ideas and how to organize ideas for recall.

   f. Provide practice listening for information with and without distracting noises such as cafeteria noise, TV or radio playing, and other students talking.

2. Materials:

   a. Checklists of listening skills.
   b. Topics to be covered by classroom teacher, with main ideas highlighted.
   c. Tapes of recorded classroom, hallway, cafeteria noises.
   d. Texts from previous classes, articles from newspapers of interest to the child/adolescent for use when reading paragraphs

5. Checklist for development of recognition of attention behaviors for self-analysis.

B. Outcome criteria: Teenager will describe self-attending abilities for the classroom that are 75% accurate according to the therapist and teacher. Teenager will appropriately ask for repeats or slowing down when important information is presented in class 75% of the time. Teenager will locate main ideas or important vocabulary with 80% accuracy. And, teenager will improve ability to concentrate on auditorially presented information in distracting conditions without becoming frustrated for up to 5 minutes.

II. Employment

A. Goal: To improve teenager's competence to follow verbal directions necessary to be successful on the job.

1. Activities:

   a. Teach vocabulary of the job.
   b. Develop sequencing abilities, both visually and auditorially.
   c. Teach compensatory strategies; note taking, repetition, re-auditorization, rehearsal, self-talk, chunking.
   d. Outline methods for requesting additional information and clarification.

2. Materials:

   a. Vocabulary and typical verbal directions obtained from employer.
   b. *Handbook of Exercises for Language Processing* (HELP) manuals II, III (Lazzari and Peters, 1980a, 1980b, 1989).
   c. *125 Ways To Be A Better Student* (Lingui-Systems)

III. Social

A. Goal: To improve child's ability to respond correctly to organizational task directed by verbal input.

1. Activities:
   a. Child/adolescent follows therapist's directions about how to complete a craft and/or play a barrier game.
   b. Learn rules for new game by listening, then doing.
   c. Use friend or parent in play situations with dolls, trucks, Legos to introduce following directions and turn taking.
   d. Bruner (1983) suggests peek-a-boo as a means of simultaneously developing deep language structure and social interactions. Peek-a-boo is not usually played the same way each time. To introduce auditory practice, call the child from various locations, give simple directions "over here," "under the table," etc. to engage auditory functioning.
2. Materials:
   a. Consult Communication Skill Builders, Speech Bin, DLM, PRO-ED, Thinking Publications, Midwest Publications catalogs for a variety of materials that can be adapted.
   b. Develop sets of crafts, games, and cards that can be adapted. See Deaton (1991) for goals, modifications, quantification, and observation examples that can be developed with games.

B. Outcome Criteria: Child will participate in games, crafts for up to 5 minutes while given only auditory directions 85% of the time with therapist and 75% of the time with significant others present.

IV. Independent Living:
   A. Goal: To increase teenager's ability to employ appropriate receptive language skills while obtaining needed information from community members.
   1. Activities:
      a. Determine what significant information needs to be obtained (time of show, price of tickets, hours of operation, location of store, rental information, means for obtaining phone installation, etc,)
      b. Organize list of questions needed to obtain all information.
      c. Rehearse questioning and answering procedures, including requesting repeats and additional information.
   2. Materials:
      a. Phone book.
      b. Newspapers, advertisements.
   B. Outcome Criteria: Teenager will understand information provided over phone or in-person about information sought 75% of the time by using receptive language skills only.

Functional Outcome-Based Plan: Expressive Language

I. School
  A. Goal: To increase ability to respond verbally to teacher requests during small group instruction in health.
    1. Activities:
      a. Teach health vocabulary and ability to name and define each word.
      b. Teach questioning procedures and how to respond to questions.
      c. Rehearse responding to questions about health lesson.
      d. Introduce strategies for sequencing, determining main ideas, themes.
      e. Rehearse verbal restatements of main ideas and themes and how to sequence responses using health lessons.
    2. Materials
      a. Health text and teacher-selected vocabulary.
      b. *125 Ways To Be a Better Student* (Lingui-Systems)
      c. Present vocabulary and have child organize by theme and how each relates to the other.
      d. Have child sequence events of the day and daily routines such as dressing, preparing for school, events in the classroom. Have child find the main idea from paragraphs in the health text being used.
      e. Playing telegram, have the child select the vocabulary that will define the health lesson in the fewest, most important words.
  B. Outcome Criteria: Child will respond verbally to teacher's questions about the health lesson with 75% accuracy using appropriate vocabulary.

III. Employment
  A. Goal: To increase ability to engage in conversational speech with customers that is concise and gains information needed to complete job.
    1. Activities:
      a. Learn expressive vocabulary and activities needed (task analysis) to complete job (such as server in a small restaurant)
      b. Rehearse conversation and activities necessary to complete the job.
      c. Role play the conversation and possible unexpected requests within the job situation.
      d. Complete the role in an actual situation, with feedback provided.

2. Materials:
   a. Vocabulary and job description.
   b. *Communication Workshop* (Zakim, 1986).
   c. Develop role play conversational scenarios developed to be employed in rehearsal.
B. Outcome Criteria: Teen will engage in appropriate conversation for job task 100% of time with therapist and 95% of time in job situation.

III. Social
A. Goal: To increase ability to engage in appropriate discussion about pertinent events with friends.
   1. Activities:
      a. Rehearse expressive vocabulary needed for conversations with friends about topics of interest.
      b. Role-play conversational situations and include unexpected changes of topic, intrusions of others, and so on.
      c. Provide exercises in topic maintenance.
      d. Provide small group conversations with peers.
      e. Ask child/adolescent to maintain a journal or diary of interactions with successes and problems in using vocabulary and topic maintenance.
   2. Materials
      a. Topics developed for conversation, such as:
         • Listen to sports commentators and develop a vocabulary of sports terms ("0 and 3," "tighten up on the bat," "can't find the plate," "base on balls," "they're trying to come alive," "a high fly ball to right field," etc.)
         • Soap opera story lines (many newspapers carry weekly summaries)
         • Listings of area malls and popular stores
         • Cosmetic items and brands popular with friends
         • Musical groups and popular songs
         • Favorite foods ordered at fast food restaurants
B. Outcome Criteria: Child will converse with friends using correct vocabulary and expressive language 80% of time in controlled situations and 70% of time in spontaneous conversational opportunities.

IV. Independent Living
A. Goal: To improve child's ability to use expressive language to express hopes, fears, wants.
   1. Activities
      a. Use pictures illustrating various emotions to establish names for different feelings.

    b. Provide atmosphere in treatment and help family also to provide atmosphere in which child is free to express hopes and fears.

    c. Use·pictures of various situations (such as picnics, family outings, families working together, children in a hospital, a child falling from a bike) to help the child use vocabulary and sentence structure to describe the activity and possible feelings surrounding the picture.

    d. Allow time for expression of emotions and hopes in each session if the child desires to discuss.

  2. Materials:

    a. Materials from catalogs such as Speech Bin, Communication Skill Builders, Interactive Therapeutics, Lingui-Systems can be adapted.

It was important for me to remind everyone that my son responded best to those who have a sense of humor. (Jason's Mom)

  B. Outcome Criteria: Child will use expressive language (both vocabulary and sentence structure) to verbally express concerns, joys, fears, 75% of time so that significant others in the environment understand these aspects of the child's life.

Functional Outcome-Based Plan: Pragmatic Language

  I. School

    A. Goal: To increase appropriate turn taking in classroom discussions.

      1. Activities:

        a. Develop ability to self-analyze skills in relationship to social rules, expectations, and routines for conversations.

        b. Develop ability to recognize communication partner's interactions, nonverbal messages, intent to maintain conversational lead.

        c. Rehearse strategies for requesting conversational turns in a classroom environment.

        d. Role play conversations and teacher/class interactions.

        e. Develop a self-monitoring and self-rewarding procedure for maintaining appropriate conversational role in the classroom.

        f. Develop a checklist or log for the child to use to monitor own classroom turn taking and practice using it. (Therapist may want to attend class discussion and make checklist to compare with child's checklist).

    2. Materials
       a. Videotapes.
       b. *Communication Workshop* (Zakim, 1986).
       c. Scripts for role play based on teacher information about what is expected in classroom discussions.
  B. Outcome Criteria: Child will self-monitor conversational turn taking and neither interrupt nor refuse to relinquish the conversation inappropriately 75% of the time within the classroom and 90% with therapist.

III. Employment
  A. Goal: To improve teenager's ability to accept constructive criticism on the job and respond with acceptable verbal behavior.
    1. Activities:
      a. Provide exposure to activities that develop executive functioning.
- Self awareness: description of personal strengths and areas for improvement.
- Goal setting: learn to set own therapy goals, determine dates for completion of tasks, keep records of accomplishments and areas for improvement.
- Planning: help therapist plan therapy or tutoring sessions.
- Initiating: allow child/adolescent to initiate activities or verbalize what should be done and then initiate.
- Inhibiting: ask for description of what went wrong, how child/adolescent could have stopped the inappropriate behavior; encourage self-talk.
- Monitoring: provide means to self-describe behaviors and suggest alterations as an activity is taking place.
- Evaluating: introduce checklists, video monitoring, employer feedback as a means of determining what was successful and unsuccessful in a job task.

      b. Include discussions of emotional and nonverbal responses when told something went wrong and offer ways to remediate on the job.
      c. Role-play conversations between teenager and employer.
      d. Rehearse and model appropriate responses to criticisms of job performance.
    2. Materials:
      a. Obtain job descriptions of expectations for performance.
      b. Video responses to criticism and analyze for what was accepted and what was not.
  B. Outcome Criteria: Teen will respond with socially appropriate verbal responses to on-the-job constructive criticism 75% of the time with employer and 90% with therapist.

IV. Social

    A. Goal: To increase ability to use humor and jokes with friends and family.

        1. Activities:

            a. Use age-appropriate cartoons, comics to establish word content and meaning and how humor applies.

            b. Develop skills with antonyms and synonyms.

            c. Write lines for blank cartoon pictures or comics.

            d. Practice slang responses and humorous answers to questions.

            e. Learn appropriate times to use slang or humor.

            f. Practice with puns, humorous responses.

            g. Use responses in structured peer interactions.

        2. Materials

            a. *Disney's Comic Strip Maker* (1988).

            b. Multiple-level comics, cartoons, jokes, and puns compilations.

            c. List of acceptable slang expressions used by peers and family.

            d. HELP manuals (Lingui-Systems)

            e. Sticky Bear: Opposites

    B. Outcome Criteria: Child will understand humor and respond with appropriate verbal responses in structured and unstructured peer conversations.

IV. Independent Living

    A. Goal: To improve abilities to advocate for self by using appropriate problem solving skills.

        1. Activities:

            a. Teach executive functioning activities.

            b. Develop causal reasoning abilities.

            c. Develop deductive and inductive reasoning skills.

            d. Develop ability to propose multiple solutions and justify the solution selected.

            e. Place in natural settings within the facility (cafeteria, bathroom, bedroom) and allow practice in problem solving (if wheel chair gets stuck in a corner of the hallway, if toilet paper is empty, if desired item in cafeteria is gone, and so on.)

            f. Rehearse conversations with potential community members to describe communication problems and help develop solutions.

        2. Materials

            a. Picture cards of hypothetical situations.

            b. Concrete problems, such as geometric puzzle pieces that fit into a ball, sticks that need to be placed to "reach" an object, and so on.

     c. Consult commercial catalogs for materials.
- **B.** Outcome Criteria: Child will verbally present problems of integrating self into a community activity to family, then community representative. Child will also contribute to development of a solution to the problem.

If We Want the Child to Fly: Integrated Approaches

We have emphasized functional application of therapy for the child/adolescent with TBI to achieve maximum potential and development. There must be an integrated approach that encompasses all aspects of daily living over the life cycle. All aspects—language, organization, memory, executive functioning, perception, and attention—are interdependent and must be considered as such in any therapeutic planning.

Otto, a father of Rachel's friend, reached out to help Jason bring out positive thoughts. Otto owns an auto repair shop that refurbishes old cars. He took Jason to work with him many times to help him gain some self-esteem, self-worth, to work hard, to listen, and talk from the heart. (Jason's Mom)

Collaboration with family, teachers, peers, community helpers affords the most integrated means of assisting the child/adolescent to become a productive adult within our society. To make that adaptation within society successful, the problems of communication and how to adapt to them must be understood.

By describing both the underlying cognitive processes and the behaviors of the individual in specific terms, a picture of how a child/adolescent with TBI may perform in functional situations can begin to emerge. Persons in the environment may begin to understand why these behaviors can occur. Problems areas may also be anticipated and described in specific terms. Interactions can focus on developing reasonable compensations for the individual within given situations. And solutions are often proposed by significant others in the environment.

To communicate clearly about cognitive-communicative impairments and how they may appear in a given environment, several steps should be taken.

1. **Describe the behavior.** Outline in specific terms what is occurring. For example, a child is daydreaming in class and the teacher describes this behavior as lack of concern, unwillingness to participate in class discussions.

2. **Determine a possible cognitive-communicative impairment that may describe why the behavior is occurring.** The child is not day-dreaming. There are two possible problems. One is that antiseizure medication is affecting concentration. The other is that the child's attention to verbal presentations is too short to maintain attention to this teacher.

3. **Develop solutions.** The therapist may work with a child to increase attention, and teach compensatory strategies. The teacher may modify personal behavior to call attention from the child when needed; the family may need to consult with the physician about effects of medication.

Appendix D is a series of charts that describe a variety of behaviors in different situations, possible cognitive-communicative impairments contributing to the behaviors, strategies that can be employed by the therapist, teacher, or family that may help alter behaviors. Resources for teaching the strategies are similar to those listed in Appendix C. Charts are developed for receptive language problems, expressive language problems, writing problems, social behaviors, and general behaviors (Blosser & DePompei, 1989). The material is intended as example and is not directed toward any age or developmental level. At the end of each table is a blank page that can be used collaboratively by family members, therapists, and teachers to develop individual descriptions and possible solutions for each child.

Making communication partners a part of the remediation of communication processes in various environments may be a vital part of the overall rehabilitation and reintegration program. Their contributions will be more effective if they use strategies they know can help and have the confidence to implement the strategies when needed. Helping them to participate with understanding and knowledge can be essential to successful reintegration and maintenance within home, school, work, or community.

Summary Guidelines

1. Treatment of cognitive-communicative disorders must be focused on the expectations for communication within home, school, work, or community life.

2. Many techniques learned for other populations with communication disorders will be appropriate to the needs of the child/adolescent with TBI.

3. Direct intervention for communication improvement must be centered in approaches that recognize different developmental levels of functioning.

4. There are differences in rehabilitation, modification, and compensation. These different processes must be recognized and used appropriately to avoid placing undue pressure on the child/adolescent to acquire skills that the youngster is not capable of developing or relearning.

5. Therapy may sometimes be discontinued to allow for normal development over time. It may also sometimes be discontinued to permit preservation of funds for later needs.

6. Although direct interventions usually focus on deficit areas, residual strengths should be employed to aid in development of self-esteem and as means for compensation.

7. All aspects of language—organization, memory, executive functioning, perception, attention, receptive and expressive skills at all levels—are interdependent and must be considered in any therapeutic planning.

8. If children/adolescents with TBI are to learn to fly, we as Merlin, must learn to take them to the edge and then let go.

References

Arvedson, J. C. (1993). Pediatric swallowing and feeding disorders. *Journal of Medical Speech-Language Pathology, 1*(4), 203–221.

Begali, V. (1987). *Head injury in children and adolescents: A resource and review for school and allied professionals.* Brandon, VT: Clinical Psychology Publishers.

Beukelman D., & Mirenda, P. (1992). *Augmentative and alternative communication: Management of severe communication disorders in children and adults.* Baltimore: Paul H. Brookes Publishing Co.

Beukelman, D. R., & Yorkston, K. (1991). *Communication disorders following traumatic brain injury: Management of cognitive, language, and motor impairments.* Austin, TX: PRO-ED.

Blosser, J. L., & DePompei, R. (1989). The head injured student returns to school: Recognizing and treating deficits. *Topics in Language Disorders, 9*(2), 67–77.

Blosser, J. L., & DePompei, R. (1992). A proactive model for treating communication disorders in children and adolescents with traumatic brain injury. *Clinics in Communicative Disorders, 2*(2), 52-65.

Bosma, J. F. (1980). Physiology of the mouth, pharynx, and esophagus. In M. Paparella & D. Shumrick (Eds.), *Otolaryngology* (2nd ed.) (pp. 319–345). Philadelphia: Saunders.

Bosma, J. F. (1986). Development of feeding. *Journal of Clinical Nutrition, 5*, 210–218.

Bosma, J. F. (1992). Development and impairments of feeding in infancy and childhood. In M. E. Groeher (Ed.), *Dysphagia: Diagnosis and management.* Boston: Butterworth-Heinemann.

Bruner, J. S. (1983). *Child's talk: Learning to use language.* New York: W.W. Norton.

Cohen, S. (1986). Educational reintegration and programming for children with head injuries. *Journal of Head Trauma Rehabilitation, 1*(2), 22–29.

Cohen, S.(1991). Adapting educational programs for students with head injuries. *Journal of Head Trauma Rehabilitation, 6*(1), 56–63.

Deaton, A. (1991). Rehabilitating cognitive impairments through the use of games. In J. S. Kreutzer & P. H. Wehman (Eds.), *Cognitive rehabilitation for persons with traumatic brain injury: A functional approach* (pp. 201–213). Baltimore: Paul H. Brookes Publishing Co.

DePompei, R., & Blosser, J. L. (1991). Functional cognitive-communicative impairments in children and adolescents: Assessment and intervention. In J. Kreutzer & P. Wehman (Eds.), *Cognitive rehabilitation for persons with traumatic brain injury.* Baltimore: Paul H. Brookes Publishing Co.

DePompei, R., & Blosser, J. L. (1993). Professional training and development for pediatric rehabilitation. In C. Durgin, N. Schmidt, & J. Freyer (Eds.), *Staff development and clinical intervention in brain injury rehabilitation* (pp. 229–253). Gaithersburg, MD: Aspen.

Deruyter, F., & Kennedy, M. (1991). Augmentative communication following traumatic brain injury. In D. R. Beukelman & K. Yorkston (Eds.), *Communication disorders following traumatic brain injury: Management of cognitive, language, and motor impairments* (pp. 317–365). Austin, TX: PRO-ED.

Gillette, Y. (1994). Early intervention in communication development: A model for professionals consulting with families. In M. Smith & J. Damico (Eds.), *Childhood language disorders.* New York: Thieme Medical Publishers.

Groher, M. (1992). (Ed.). *Dysphagia: Diagnosis and management.* Boston: Butterworth-Heinemann.

Jones, B. (Ed.) *Dysphagia.* NY: Springer-Verlag.

Hagen, C. (1988). Treatment of aphasia: A process approach. *Journal of Head Trauma Rehabilitation, 3*(2), 23–34.

Kaslon, K., & Ruben, R. J. (1978). Traumatically acquired conditioned dysphagia in children. *Annals of Otology Rhinology and Laryngology, 87*, 509–514.

Kenny, D. J., Kohiel, R. M., & Greenberg, J. (1989). Development of a multidisciplinary feeding program for children who are dependent feeders. *Dysphagia 4*, 16–28.

Kennedy, M., & Deruyter, F. (1991). Cognitive and language bases for communication disorders. In D. R. Beukelman & K. M. Yorkston (Eds.), *Communication disorders following traumatic brain injury: Management of cognitive, language, and motor impairments* (pp. 123–190). Austin, TX: PRO-ED.

Kilpatrick, K. (1976). *Therapy guide for adults with language and speech disorders.* Akron, OH: Visiting Nurse Service.

Kilpatrick, K., & DePompei, R. (1986). *Working with words on your own.* Akron, OH: Visiting Nurse Service.

Klein, P. S. (1981). Nutritional deprivation and retardation of cognitive functions. In P. Mittler (Ed.), *Frontiers of knowledge of mental retardation*, vol. 2, Biomedical aspects (pp. 121–142.). Baltimore: University Park Press.

Kraat, A., & Sitver-Kogut, M. (1993). *Features of portable communication devices.* Wilmington, DE: Applied Science & Engineering Laboratories.

Kreutzer, J. (1993, April). *Community reintegration: Assessment concerns.* Presentation at St John's Medical Center, Detroit, MI.

Kreutzer, J. S., & Wehman, P. H. (1991). *Cognitive rehabilitation for persons with traumatic brain injury.* Baltimore: Paul H. Brookes Publishing Co.

Lash, M., & Wolcott, G. (in press). *When your teenager is injured: Moving from school to work.* Boston: Exceptional Parent.

Langfitt, T., & Gennarelli, T. (1982). Can outcome from head injury be improved? *Journal of Neurosurgery, 56,* 19–25.

Lazarus, C. (1991). Diagnosis and management of swallowing disorders in traumatic brain injury. In D. R. Beukelman & K. M. Yorkston (Eds.), *Communication disorders following traumatic brain injury: Management of cognitive, language, and motor impairments* (pp. 367–417). Austin, TX: PRO-ED.

Lazarus, C., & Logemann, J. (1987). Swallowing disorders in closed head trauma patients. *Archives of Physical Medicine and Rehabilitation, 68,* 79–84.

Lazzari, A., & Peters, P. M. (1980a). *HELP: Handbook of exercises for language processing, Volume I.* Moline, IL: Lingui-Systems.

Lazzari, A., & Peters, P. M. (1980b). *HELP: Handbook of exercises for language processing, Volume II.* Moline, IL: Lingui-Systems.

Lazzari, A., & Peters, P. M. (1989a). *HELP: Handbook of exercises for language processing, Volume III.* Moline, IL: Lingui-Systems.

Lazzari, A., & Peters, P. M. (1989b). *HELP: Handbook of exercises for language processing, Volume IV.* Moline, IL: Lingui-Systems.

Logemann, J. (1983). *Evaluation and treatment of swallowing disorders.* Boston: College-Hill Press.

Marquardt, T. P., & Sussman, H. M. (1991). Developmental apraxia of speech: Theory and practice. In D. Vogel & M. P. Cannito (Eds.), *Treating disordered speech motor control. For clinicians by clinicians.* Austin, TX: PRO-ED.

Milton, S. B. (1988). Management of subtle cognitive communicative deficits. *Journal of Head Trauma Rehabilitation, 3*(2), 1–11.

Milton, S., Scaglione, C., Flanagan, T., Cox, J. L., & Rudnick, D. (1991). Functional evaluation of adolescent students with traumatic brain injury. *Journal of Head Trauma Rehabilitation, 6*(2), 35–46.

Mollitt, D. L., Golladay, E. S., & Seibert, J. J. (1985). Symptomatic gastroesophageal reflux following gastrostomy in neurologically impaired patients. *Pediatrics, 75,* 1124–1126.

Morris, S. E. (1989). Development of oral-motor skills in the neurologically impaired child receiving non-oral feedings. *Dysphagia, 3,* 135–154.

Morris, S. E., & Klein, M. D. (1987). *Pre-feeding skills. A comprehensive resource for feeding development.* Tucson, AZ: Communication Skill Builders.

Parenté, R., & Anderson, J. K. (1983). Techniques for improving cognitive rehabilitation: Teaching organization and encoding skills. *Cognitive Rehabilitation, 1*(4), 20–22.

Parenté, R., & DiCesare, J. (1991). Retraining memory: Theory, evaluation and applications. In J. S. Kreutzer & P. H. Wehman (Eds.), *Cognitive rehabilitation for persons with traumatic brain injury* (pp. 147–162). Baltimore: Paul H. Brookes Publishing Co.

Patrick, J., & Geisel, E. G. (1990). Nutrition for the neurologically impaired child. *Journal of Neurology Rehabilitation, 4*, 115–119.

Rosenthal, M., & Berrol, S. (1989). Swallowing disorders and rehabilitation. *Journal of Head Trauma Rehabilitation, 4*(4), 1–92.

Rosenwinkel-Marsalla, P. (1983–1989). *Innovative concepts: Speech and language therapy newsletter.* Seattle: Innovative Concepts.

Russell, N. (1993). Educational considerations in traumatic brain injury: The role of the speech/language pathologist. *Language, Speech, and Hearing Services in the Schools, 24*(2), 67–75.

Sanford, J. A., & Browne, R. J. (1985). *Captain's log: Cognitive training system, visual/motor skills module, visual tracking/discrimination* (computer program). Richmond, VA: Network Services.

Smith, J. (1984). *Cognitive rehabilitation* (computer program). Diamondale, MI: Hartley Courseware, Inc.

Sohlberg, M. M., & Mateer, C. A. (1987). *Attention process training (APT).* Puyallup, WA: Association for Neuropsychological Research and Development.

Sohlberg, M. M., & Mateer, C. A. (1989). The assessment of cognitive-communicative functions in head injury. *Topics in Language Disorders, 9*(2), 15–33.

Telzrow, C. F. (1987). Management of academic and educational problems in head injury. *Journal of Learning Disabilities, 20*, 536–545.

Telzrow, C. F. (1994). Best practices in facilitating intervention adherence. In A. Thomas & J. Grimes (Eds.), *Best practices in school psychology.* Washington, DC: National Association of School Pyschologists.

Wehman, P. (1992). *Life beyond the classroom: Transition strategies for young people with disabilities.* Baltimore: Paul H. Brookes Publishing Co.

Wilson, J. M. (1977). *Oral-motor function and dysfunction in children.* Chapel Hill, NC: University of North Carolina at Chapel Hill, Division of Physical Therapy.

Yorkston, K., & Beukelman, D. (1991). Motor speech disorders. In D. R. Beukelman & K. Yorkston (Eds.), *Communication disorders following traumatic brain injury: Management of cognitive, language, and motor impairments.* Austin, TX: PRO-ED.

Ylvisaker, M.(1985). *Head injury rehabilitation: Children and adolescents.* San Diego: College-Hill Press.

Ylvisaker, M. (1993). *Assessment and treatment of traumatic brain injury with school age children and adults.* Buffalo, NY:EDUCOM

Ylvisaker, M., Chorazy, A., Cohen, S., Mastrill, J., Molitor, C., Nelson, J., Sezekeres, S., Valko, A., & Jaffe, K. (1990). Rehabilitative assessment following head injury in children. In M. Rosenthal, E. Griffeth, M. Bond, & J. D. Miller (Eds.), *Rehabilitation of the adult and child with traumatic brain injury* (2nd ed.) (pp. 558–584). Philadelphia: F. A. Davis.

Zakim, S. (1986). *Communication workshop.* E. Moline, IL: Lingui-Systems.

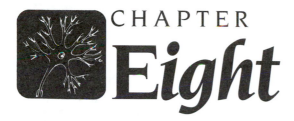

CHAPTER

Eight

Modifying the Communication Environment

Direct treatment to teach a youngster new and compensatory communication strategies is essential. However, we cannot expect a child to bear all of the responsibility for making changes. People who live, work, play with, and teach the child can learn to modify the environment and their own communication patterns and styles to provide support and assistance to a child. First, all must realize the influence their communicative interaction has on a child's performance. Difficulties that may occur during problematic communicative interactions may lead to a communication breakdowns, frustration, and even punishment for the child.

The third family conference had nine individuals from the rehab team, school, insurance company, Tom, and I. It was determined that it would be beneficial to have a homebound teacher work with my son in addition to the academics teacher at the Rehab Center. Once again, the "senses" of a Mom had to come into play. The initial teacher they assigned to my son had a heavy accent. Recognizing that he had a low concentration level, short attention span, and problems expressing new ideas, I knew that the last thing he needed was someone he couldn't understand. (Jason's Mom)

People who are important in the child's life can easily learn to incorporate critical communication modification strategies into home routines, teaching lessons, work coaching, and social exchanges. These strategies can help increase a youngster's potential for understanding others, following directions, and communicating more effectively (Blosser, 1990; Blosser & DePompei, 1992b, DePompei & Blosser, 1992).

In this chapter, the reader will learn to:

1. Identify significant people in the youngster's environment who can participate meaningfully in the treatment process.

2. Recognize the communication manners and styles of other individuals that may interfere with the youngster's success.

3. Select the appropriate interaction and instructional strategies to teach the significant people in the youngster's world.

4. Determine procedures for teaching the selected techniques to others.

Doable Strategies for Communication Partners

It is as important for clinicians to provide direct instruction to a child's significant communication partners (relatives, friends, teachers, work associates) as it is to work directly with the child; perhaps even more important, because it is through their efforts that the child's new behaviors will become solidified. The problem the clinician faces is deciding who to involve, what strategies to teach them, and how to convey the information. Care has to be taken to explain the recommended methods clearly, eliminating professional jargon from the discussion. It is also wise to recommend only a limited number of effective communication modification strategies. Otherwise, the task will become too complicated and overwhelming. Careful selection of strategies suggested to others should be based on the nature of a youngster's injury; the assessment of cognitive-communicative processes; descriptions of the demands and expectations for performance in particular environmental contexts; and, the communication partner's interactive communication style. Several factors that should be considered when recommending strategies for interaction are:

1. The relationship of the helper to the person with TBI;

2. The severity of the communication impairment;

3. The communication partner's general knowledge about characteristics of TBI;

4. The individual's willingness to try to modify communicative interactions with the child;

5. Time available and commitment to participating in the process;

6. The helper's ability to understand and provide meaningful assistance; and,

7. The circumstances of the interactions the person will have with the youngster.

Steps to the Edge

The process others must learn involves three steps: (1) recognizing when the youngster is experiencing difficulty as a result of cognitive-communication impairments; (2) understanding the underlying impairment that is causing a behavior; and (3) making a change in the communication environment or manner and style of communication with the youngster that will facilitate a better performance by the child. This means that the people with whom the child interacts most frequently must learn to be astute observers and reporters. They must develop an understanding of the child's disability and the impact it has on performance. Most importantly, they must learn to recognize which of their own interactive communication mannerisms and styles serves to facilitate positive responses or create problems. This will help others realize that they have the power to bring the situation under better control by modifying their own communication manner and style.

Observe the Youngster's Behaviors

People who are around the child with TBI have ample opportunities to observe problematic and inappropriate behaviors. In fact, when conferring with parents and teachers about a child, the discussion will quite often include explanations of specific situations that occurred or something that happened to the child. For example, "he kept telling the same jokes over and again—his friends got bored and left"; "he talks too loud, others are embarrassed to go out in public with him"; "she never seems to remember the directions for doing her homework—the teacher gives her Fs on all of her work"; "she always interrupts others when they are talking—I can tell it irritates them." Comments such as these deserve attention and further investigation. They can form the basis for developing a better understanding of the child's problems and needs. More importantly, they can provide opportunity for identifying steps that can be taken to provide support to the child.

Relate the Observed Behavior to an Underlying Cognitive-Communicative Impairment

When our evaluations of children are complete, we generally construct a written or verbal report describing the strengths and weaknesses. Many times, these are presented to others as a "laundry list" of behaviors: "as a result of the TBI, her speech is slurred; she has difficulty learning new information; she can't efficiently process information she hears; she isn't able to express her thoughts very clearly." Some clinicians go a step further and give one or two examples of how the deficit might look in real-life situations. These clinicians are on the right track. They are laying the groundwork for helping others understand the child better. The next step is to develop the communication partners' capability to relate the child's performance in particular situations to one of the "laundry list" impairments. This can be facilitated by listening attentively as the situations are described and helping the partner sort through the list, trying to match a behavior to the impairment. For example, the situations mentioned above might be related to the child's inability to recognize nonverbal cues, monitor voice loudness, identify when important information such as directions are being given, and take turns during conversations.

Modify Communication Manner and Style in Response to the Youngster's Strengths and Needs

When a child/adolescent has difficulty, support needs to be provided at that moment. The communication partner needs to respond quickly to help alter the course of the situation. Selected individuals who live, teach, go to school, play, and work with a student can assume meaningful roles in communication rehabilitation, if permitted to do so. Unfortunately, well-meaning persons occasionally end up interfering with success because of their misperceptions about the cause of the student's behavior and their own communicative interaction with the child. It would be better if the communication partner understood how to elicit specific types of positive responses from a child and to seize opportunities for providing assistance. Family members, teachers, friends, and co-workers need to develop a repertoire of communicative strategies they can try to turn the situations into more positive directions.

A foundation must be laid to help others understand these concepts. First, they must recognize their own interactive communication manner and style. Next, they must understand the effect their style may be having on a child's performance. Finally, they must take steps to make a change in their own behavior to bring about effective change in the child's performance. Guided discussion and questioning techniques can be used to convey this process to others and to help them understand the influence their own communicative behavior has on the youngster. Providing descriptive examples will also help enlighten others: "Johnny needs a longer period of time to think about what he has heard before he can come up with answers to questions. He will especially have difficulty if the person he talks to uses a fast rate of speech. If you ask the question slowly and let him take time to think, I'll bet he'll give you better answers." If this example is being conveyed to a person who speaks very rapidly, most likely a "light will go off" and the person will realize the effect their own behavior may be having on a child's performance.

The procedures for assessing the environment and people in the child's environment described in Chapter 6 can be used to establish the basis for planning the specific strategies to teach others. (See Table 6–3, "The Communication Style Identification Chart, page 132).

To be functional, the child should practice new skills throughout the day and in informal, natural contexts. Informal communicative interactions and classroom instructional activities can offer unique opportunities for skill development. Clinicians and therapists are not the appropriate individuals to carry out this charge. Rather, family, teachers, peers, and co-workers can implement practice strategies during ongoing interactions with a child.

Strategies That Can Be Recommended To Others

Table 8–1, "Planning Interactive Cognitive-Communication Modification Strategies," illustrates numerous interactive communication strategies others can learn to implement for providing support to a child when needed to improve or correct the quality of performance. The professional plays an important role in helping select the appropriate strategy. Time should be spent explaining the communication strategy to significant communicators in a child's life and helping them understand how to match a communication strategy to the behaviors observed.

Strategies such as these have been helpful with children and adolescents who exhibit cognitive-communication impairments as a result of TBI. Care should be taken in selecting specific strategies. Not all are appropriate for all children. The strategies should not all be used (or taught) simultaneously. Rather, the clinician should strive to **match the strategy and make modifications to meet the child's individualized needs**

Table 8-1. Planning interactive cognitive-communication modification strategies.

This outline of cognitive-communication strategies can be used while interacting with and teaching students with traumatic brain injury. Following formal and informal assessment procedures, check those cognitive-communication strategies to be implemented and/or modified when interacting with or teaching the student.

For example, use Monitoring Quality of Conversations, if assessment revealed that the student has difficulty understanding long, complex sentences. The communication partners should make attempts to modify their communication styles by using short, simple sentences and reducing sentence complexity.

Monitoring Quality of Conversations
____ Reduce length of utterances
____ Reduce complexity of utterances
____ Reduce rate of speech
____ Vary voice patterns
____ Vary intonation patterns to emphasize key words

Giving Instructions and Directions
____ Reduce length of instructions
____ Reduce complexity of instructions
____ Reduce rate of delivery
____ Repeat instructions more than once
____ Alter mode of instruction delivery
____ Give prompts and assistance

Explaining New Concepts and Vocabulary
____ Give definitions for terms
____ Show visual representations of concepts and vocabulary
____ Give definitions for terms
____ Show visual representations of concepts and vocabulary
____ Present only a restricted number of new concepts at a time
____ Ask questions to be sure of understanding

Monitoring Speech Selection
____ Avoid sarcasm
____ Avoid idiomatic expressions
____ Limit humor
____ Avoid puns

Organizing and Sequencing Information
____ Present information in clusters and groups
____ Introduce information with attention-getting words

Attending to Student's Behaviors, Queries, Comments
____ Redirect behaviors
____ Reinforce queries and appropriate behaviors and comments
____ Select material appropriate for skill, age, interest

Supporting Verbal Communication
_____ Use or reduce gestures dependent on student response
_____ Use visual clues
_____ Incorporate imagery to increase understanding

Permitting Adequate Response Time
_____ Provide ample time for responses

Announcing and Clarifying Topic of Conversation
_____ Introduce the topic to be discussed
_____ Restate topic of discussion

Making the Student Aware of Others' Responses
_____ Inform student of verbal signs and their meaning
_____ Inform student of nonverbal signs and their meaning

Reading to the Student
_____ Reduce rate
_____ Reduce length
_____ Reduce complexity
_____ Determine comprehension through questioning
_____ Redirect student's attention to important details and facts

Communicating Through Writing
_____ Evaluate quality
_____ Provide ample time for task completion
_____ Evaluate accuracy
_____ Assist with organizational structure
_____ Guide changes in legibility and structure

Reinforcing the Student's Communication Attempts
_____ Redirect so responses are pragmatically appropriate
_____ Inform student if message is not understandable
_____ Model correct productions
_____ Correct error productions

Requiring and Expecting Communication
_____ Provide communication opportunities

Encouraging Responsiveness
_____ Have the student re-read instructions and material
_____ Ask the student to repeat instructions and information to ensure understanding
_____ Guide student through proofreading work
_____ Assist student in evaluating quality of work and accomplishments

(continues)

Table 8–1. (*continued*)

_____

Fostering Communication Through any Means Possible
_____ Introduce alternative/augmentative communication systems

Arranging the Physical Environment for Communication
_____ Reduce distractions
_____ Eliminate physical barriers
_____ Guide student in understanding appropriate proximity

Structuring Communication Activities
_____ Provide opportunities for group interactions
_____ Vary group size
_____ Vary composition of group
_____ Vary formality of interaction opportunities

Developing Memory Skills
_____ Encourage student to categorize information
_____ Encourage student to make associations
_____ Provide opportunities for rehearsing information
_____ Assist student in visualizing information
_____ Encourage student to chunk information

Practicing Higher-Level Thinking and Communicating
_____ Provide opportunities for problem solving
_____ Provide opportunities for decision making
_____ Provide opportunities for making judgments
_____ Ask questions to elicit solutions, judgments, decisions

Welcoming Discussion of Frustrations, Concerns, Problems
_____ Invite open discussion

_____

based on behaviors and characteristics exhibited. Selections depend on such factors as the level of severity of the impairment, the combination of impairments, the remaining strengths and needs, the skills identified as "avenues for success," the skills targeted for improvement, the relationship of the helper to the child, the helper's capabilities for making modifications and providing assistance, and the circumstances of the interactions.

The best way clinicians can develop a list of strategies to teach to others is to closely observe and self-evaluate their own clinical techniques when working with a client. By doing this, clinicians can identify the subtle steps they take to elicit a better response or improve the quality of responses. For example, a clinician might alter voice intonation to encourage a child to do the same when the youngster's voice is too loud.

Clinicians often automatically implement subtle strategies to alter a client's performance. This is why a client's performance is often better within the structured setting of the therapy room, but slow to transfer to the home, school, community, or work setting. Several examples can be used to illustrate subtle "intuitive" steps clinicians take in response to their client's performance such as: quietly pointing to a picture to elicit a response, altering voice intonation to encourage a child to pay closer attention to a task or to listen more closely to instructions, reducing the complexity of instructions in response to a frustrated or confused look on the youngster's face, or automatically slowing speech when conveying important information or instructions.

The following brief explanation of several cognitive-communicative interaction strategies can serve as a examples of the type of information that should be conveyed when encouraging others to try to alter their manner and style of communication.

1. Monitor the Quality of Communications. Many children who sustain a TBI experience impaired comprehension skills and problems processing information presented at a fast rate. The speaker's rate of speech and quality of speech patterns can affect the child's ability to comprehend the full message. The speaker should **modify (reduce and simplify) the length, complexity, and rate of speech to accommodate the child's needs.** This means that important information, such as directions, should be expressed with shorter, less complex sentences and at a purposefully slowed rate of speech. The speaker should **vary voice and intonation patterns** when making key points.

2. Provide Instructions and Directions. A child's ability to perform required tasks and participate in activities is often dependent on the ability to accurately follow instructions. The quality and style of speaking used to deliver instructions can greatly affect a child's performance. Important instructions should be **repeated more than once and delivered via a variety of learning channels (auditory, visual, kinesthetic).** Children with severe deficits need a greater amount of modification by the speaker. The use of visual cues such as pictures, pointing, combining written instructions and spoken instructions, listing instructions in 1-2-3 order, and prompting facilitates better understanding of instructions.

3. Explain New Concepts and Vocabulary. One of the most significant problems experienced by children with TBI is the difficulty in trying to learn new information. Oftentimes, speakers imbed new concepts into discussions. It is more helpful to have a new concept highlighted for the child. This can be accomplished by defining and explaining new words or concepts as presented, using visual representations when possible. The number of concepts presented at a given time should be limited to only a few. The speaker should provide multiple opportunities for hearing, using, or understanding a new concept by repeating it in a variety of contexts. Recall of the concept can be stimulated by asking the child to recall important facts and concepts.

4. Monitor Selection of Words, Expressions, and Comments. As a result of TBI, some children have difficulty understanding common colloquial expressions and abstract comments. They can have difficulty understanding sarcasm, idioms, puns, humor, and jokes. The use of these types of language is common during social interactions. In fact, some teachers adopt such styles of speech, because the informality works well with the children they teach. However, abstract language mechanisms such as these can lead to difficulties for children with TBI when used in a classroom or as a means of trying to convey important information in a home or work setting. During informal communicative interactions with the child, these expressions should be followed with an explanation of meaning or clarification (especially if the child appears to misunderstand the comment). Use should be avoided if the topics being discussed are critical to the child's safety, learning, or understanding.

5. Organize and sequence information. Children with TBI can have difficulty understanding information presented out of context and in a random manner. Conversations that take place in informal situations are often very spontaneous and not well organized. The child's conversational partners need to be aware that this type of interchange may confuse the child. The youngster may lose track of the topic being discussed or key points being made. Therefore, it is suggested that important information be presented in a clear, organized, and sequential format. This can be accomplished by clustering information or presenting it in small segments to help draw the child's attention to important information. Beginning sentences with attention-getting words such as "first," "next," and so on will also provide assistance.

6. Attend to the youngster's behaviors, queries, and comments. People are often not attentive to a youngster's nonverbal behaviors and subtle comments. They often ignore them or do not respond. This can be observed in many exchanges that take place between children and adults. Perhaps one of the most important skills to be taught to important people in a child's life is the skill of understanding the meaning of specific behaviors and compensating for weaknesses presented by the child. Helpers can learn to observe, identify, and interpret each behavior and respond quickly and appropriately. For example, if a youngster's nonverbal behavior represents confusion or misunderstanding, changes should be made in the mode or format of presentation. Additional cues and support should be provided. If the child becomes distracted or disengaged in a conversation or activity, steps should be undertaken to redirect attention. Systems of nonverbal signals to cue the youngster to alter behavior can be prearranged and used when necessary. Some examples include calling the child's name, touching the arm, or signaling with a hand gesture. High-interest materials and reinforcement strategies also help.

7. Announce and clarify the topic of conversation. The potential for successfully navigating a conversation will be increased if a child is aware of the topic being discussed. Because attention or memory problems are often prevalent in persons with TBI, topics may get lost. Speakers should strive to introduce (or announce) a topic and restate it frequently throughout a discussion. This is especially important during classroom lectures.

8. Permit adequate response time. Conversations and classroom discussions generally move very rapidly from one speaker to the next and from topic to topic. This interaction style may prove to be very frustrating for the child with TBI. By the time thoughts are organized and responses are formulated, it is likely the conversation will have moved into another direction and additional topics will be introduced. Communication partners should be made aware of these difficulties and learn to purposefully control the pace of discussions to account for the child's processing time needs.

9. Support verbal communication. Because of the pace, organizational format, or vocabulary used, some children may have difficulty processing all information presented. Incorporating gestures, visual cues, and imagery into conversations can often enhance what is being said verbally. When using supportive communication techniques such as these, care must be taken so that they do not become distracting. Often verbal messages will be better understood if the communication partner points to objects being discussed or accompanies explanations with notes or pictures.

10. Make the child/adolescent aware of others' responses. Children with TBI are often oblivious to the mannerisms, responses, and reactions of others. If this is the case, there will be no attempt to try to make changes. Youngsters should be taught to watch other people's reactions and identify signs indicating responses such as lack of interest, boredom, and confusion and so on. This should be done cautiously and in situations that will not result in embarrassment. Showing and discussing videotapes of communication interactions may provide some insights and understanding.

11. Develop communication through writing. In school and work situations, important information is conveyed through written communication. Quality, speed, accuracy, organization, legibility, and space planning all might be affected. Therefore, it is important that written communication activities be suited to a youngster's performance capabilities in terms of structure and complexity. There are many activities that will encourage the development of children's written communication performance, including dictating sentences and facts, providing written questions to answers, and helping develop simple essays and scripts.

12. Encourage responsiveness. Children with TBI can be encouraged to use several strategies to increase their potential for more accurate performance in learning in interactive situations. These include re-reading written directions more than once, repeating verbal instructions verbatim and with paraphrasing, proofreading written work to detect errors, evaluating the success and quality of communicative efforts, and asking questions when confused about instructions. Some children cannot respond to direct questioning. In these cases, caution should be exercised when asking questions. Queries can be reframed, using directives such as "Tell me more" and "How many did you see?" If presented in association with a specific context such as a story, WH questions ("who," "what," "where," "why," "when," "how") can help facilitate development of organized communication skills. Asking leading questions can help a child identify problems and plan out solutions.

13. Require and expect communication. Often family members and friends will unknowingly convey negative messages to the child that imply they are not interested in interacting. This may be because communication is a laborious process or because the resulting interaction is embarrassing for family, friends, and others to witness. Regardless of the reason, interactive communication should be encouraged (at whatever level possible and through whatever means possible). It is via the channels of communication that modification and progress can take place. The requirements, expectations, and demands placed on a child need to be commensurate with actual capabilities.

14. Reinforce communication attempts. It is important to provide a child with feedback regarding the accuracy and quality of communication attempts. The individual should be made aware of whether or not communication attempts are pragmatically appropriate for a situation, fully understood, or produced coherently. By doing this, assistance and guidance for improving communication skills can be given. All persons working with a child should be made aware of what can realistically be expected and how to tactfully correct inappropriate behaviors and communication errors. Explaining and modeling correct behavior may be helpful, as long as explanations are simple. Confrontation and lengthy attempts at reasoning with a child with TBI should be avoided. Those actions only serve to foster a sense of failure by all people involved.

15. Encourage communication through any means possible. Children left with severe communication disabilities as a result of their TBI often cannot communicate through verbal means. Alternative or augmentative methods of communication should be introduced as early as possible to decrease the child's level of frustration and increase opportunities for interaction with others and learning. Waiting for "normal" verbal speech patterns to return or emerge can waste valuable time. Clinicians should involve family members in understanding and using alternative methods of communication to promote acceptance and maximum function of the chosen system. This suggestion applies to the application of tape recorders, calculators, computers, and assistive listening devices for facilitating achievement of classroom tasks.

16. Arrange the physical environment to encourage communication. Distractions, physical barriers, and inappropriately close proximity can all interfere with the communication process. When these situations are observed, modifications should be made. Sometimes this means removing visual and auditory distractions, rearranging objects or furniture, changing positions, or reducing the number of persons engaged in a discussion.

17. Construct communication opportunities. As a result of the length of time and design of physical recuperation following TBI, children are often away from their family and peers for long periods of time. In combination with disabilities, this can prove devastating, when it is time for the child to resume social relationships and interactions. Throughout the physical recuperation and reintegration process, group interactions ranging from very informal to formal should be arranged, so that opportunities for communication can be developed. The size, composition, and formality of a group can be modified as a child's skills strengthen. In the initial stages, it is wise to limit conversations and interactions to a few intimate family members and close friends. Over time, experience with larger, more complex groups should be encouraged. Once a child is reintegrated into home, school, and community settings, extracurricular activities should be regularly planned and scheduled. To make encounters effective, all persons involved will need to gain insights into the child's cognitive-communicative problems and behaviors. They need to learn strategies for responding to the child's behaviors and encouraging communication.

My son is very fortunate to have girls as friends. Heidi has talked to him every day since the accident, even when he was in the coma. She introduced him to two other young ladies by telephone. Thank goodness for phones and friends. (Jason's Mom)

---

18. Improve memory skills. The inability to remember assignments and previous communications proves to be extremely frustrating for a child with TBI and others with whom the youngster is communicating. Teaching techniques such as categorizing, associating, rehearsing, visualizing, and chunking information should provide assistance in improving memory skills.

19. **Practice higher level thinking and communicating.** Often children with TBI present adequate communication skills for everyday interactions, but have difficulty when the complexity of the thinking task increases. The type of assistance to provide to children who have memory problems is dictated by ability levels. In general, children should first be confronted with simple situations related to their own experiences. The difficulty level and relationship to other more far-removed situations should be gradually increased as improvement is observed. Through directive questioning, the child should be asked to explain answers and provide rationale and reasons for beliefs. This can be practiced especially well during excursions through the community when unexpected circumstances arise.

20. **Welcome discussion of frustrations, concerns, and problems.** Children with TBI suffer great frustrations. Open discussion about feelings and experiences should be encouraged so that problems can be properly handled.

Instructional Strategies

A number of instructional strategies can be recommended to educators. The strategies selected and role of an educator in implementing them should be thoroughly discussed and expressed in writing on the treatment plan. Several examples of teaching strategies that have been helpful with children with TBI are listed in Table 8–2. (The list is not meant to be exhaustive. Rather, it is provided to illustrate the concepts discussed in this section.) The same strategies, modified to suit a situation, can also be introduced to employers and leaders of community organizations.

These strategies are divided into four categories: **teacher-to-student interactional instruction strategies, student-to-student interactional instruction strategies, classroom adaptation and modification techniques, and student learning techniques (see Table 8–2).** Many more could be added to each list. By suggesting examples such as these during planning meetings, other ideas will be generated. For each strategy, the question should be asked: "Will this tactic promote opportunities for better learning and understanding for this child?" Many of the strategies, especially the student learning techniques, can be made a part of home-based programming or vocational training if family members and work coaches are provided with instruction regarding how to implement them (Blosser & DePompei, 1992; DePompei & Blosser, 1992).

Table 8–2. Instructional strategies found to be successful with students with TBI.

Teacher-to-Student Interactional Instructional Strategies

- Establish and clarify expectations for the student.
- Analyze the demands made upon the student by assigned tasks.
- Prioritize learning goals and tasks.
- Introduce information at a level that is commensurate with the youngster's developmental and mental capabilities.
- Individualize assignments and tests to accommodate special needs (reduce the number of questions, tape record lectures, increase print size, modify the format or mode of response).
- Allow multiple opportunities for practice.
- Provide feedback and guidance to increase understanding of successful and nonsuccessful attempts.
- Observe and measure performance frequently and systematically. Use information gleaned to modify teaching approaches.
- Provide incentives and consequences to stimulate motivation.
- Teach the student to recognize and measure personal success.
- Plan a specific time for rest and emotional release.
- Encourage the discussion and sharing of problems the child may be experiencing. Help the child understand the relationship between the TBI and problems occurring.
- Discuss why some of the student's behaviors are inappropriate and make suggestions for changing behavior.
- Be observant of stresses placed on the child by others (teachers, peers, family, administrators). Reduce stresses as much as possible.
- Implement holistic approaches to teaching content, involving the student actively in learning activities.

Student-to-Student Interactional Instruction Strategies

- Use cooperative learning strategies.
- Facilitate informal interactions and peer tutoring and modeling by providing small group activities.
- Select a fellow student to act as a "buddy" to help the youngster travel throughout school and participate in school-related activities.
- Select a "peer coach" to help the child remain aware of instructions, transitions from activity to activity, assignments, and so on.
- Directly teach peers to implement specific interactive communication strategies, so they are prepared to provide models and facilitate positive responses when the child with TBI exhibits difficulty or need.
- Encourage friendships and sharing through extracurricular activities based on the child's physical and emotional capabilities, interests, and so on.

(continues)

Table 8–2. (continued)

Classroom Adaptations and Modification Techniques

- Encourage the use of assistive devices, including calculators, computers, tape recorders, assistive listening devices, and so on.
- Formulate a system to help the child maintain organization (schedule book, assignment notebook, "to do" lists, and so on).
- Accompany textbooks and work pages with supportive materials (pictures, written cues, graphic illustrations, and so on).

Student Learning Techniques

- Encourage the student to **re-read** instructions more than one time, exercising care to underline, highlight, and note important elements.
- Ask the student to **repeat instructions verbatim**, before initiating a learning task.
- Verify the student's comprehension of directions by requesting that the instructions be **restated** using different terminology.
- Have the student **review** work after completing it, proofreading assignments before submission, looking for completeness and accuracy.
- Provide the student with opportunities to **repeat assignments** at another time to see if performance can be improved.
- Invite the student to **ask questions** and to **clarify information** not understood.
- Have the student **write instructions** on a separate sheet of paper.
- Have the student **self-evaluate work** to see if it is appropriate, verbalizing correct and incorrect aspects of the work.

Teacher-Student Instructional Strategies

Teachers are confronted daily by challenges posed by the diversity of students in today's schools. To meet these challenges, most teachers become very resourceful and develop a number of teaching strategies for various situations they encounter. When a child with TBI is placed in the school situation, teachers should be helped to identify those communication modification and instructional strategies that can be used to encourage the most positive learning response from the child. In addition, it is important that educators learn to identify exactly when to implement the strategy.

Student-to-Student Interactional Instruction Activities

Peer tutoring has been a successful teaching tool for improving the skills of children with disabilities. Preparing peers to play important roles in providing support and help to a classmate with TBI is paramount to successful reintegration. Time should be taken to develop peers' awareness of their fellow student's problems and establishing student-to-student interactional instructional situations.

Classroom Adaptations and Modifications

The physical, social, and teaching climate can positively or negatively affect a child's success in the learning situation. Consequently, specific adaptations that will make learning more efficient or effective should be identified and incorporated.

Student Learning Techniques

Children with TBI often experience difficulty because they are unaware of problems they have made and lack the skills to implement the changes needed at the time they are needed to improve their own performance. Asking children with learning difficulties to simply "try harder" or "do better" at learning tasks is generally as ineffective with this group of children as it is for other populations. Unfortunately, there is not always a clear link between effort and success. This is further complicated because TBI often interferes with initiative and motivation. A more proactive approach is to provide youngsters with concrete strategies for improving their own performance. This provides students with the internal resources needed to make problem-solving efforts successful. It permits some sense of control.

The ability to self-evaluate and self-monitor one's own performance is essential if learning potential is to be achieved. Research with children with learning disabilities has shown that teaching self-regulation skills is particularly helpful for children who are described as inattentive, easily distractible, and off-task during classroom activities (Licht, 1983; Reid & Harris, 1993). Teaching students to use problem-solving strategies for specific learning tasks such as writing has also been a successful teaching approach for children with disabilities (Stevens & Englert, 1993).

We visited relatives in Indiana for Easter. When we got back home, something inside positive happened to Jason and he decided to begin to become a member of the team. (Jason's Mom)

Direct emphasis in treatment for TBI should include teaching the student to initiate specific strategies to check and change self-performance of classroom work and when problematic situations occur in social interactions. It is not enough to simply teach strategies; the child must learn to relate the successful outcome of his or her performance to the use of a strategy. For this procedure to be effective, clinicians can take several steps. First, the student-learning strategies that will be most useful for a child must be identified. Second, as part of the training process, the youngster should be taught to state what the strategy is and how it did (or can) lead to improved performance. This can be accomplished by modeling the strategy for the child during a teaching interaction through self-talk or inner dialogue. (The clinician or teacher talks about what is being done as the person is doing it during the completion of a task. This may be presented to the child as "thinking out loud about what to do.") Student learning can most reliably be used in association with work assignments from the classroom setting or job assignments. (Those illustrated in Table 8–2 are merely examples of strategies that can be used to improve a student's work performance on school-related tasks.)

Additional suggestions for selecting and applying these types of strategies to meet individual student's needs are illustrated in the charts in Appendix D. Those charts illustrate the likely match between a youngster's classroom behaviors and cognitive-communicative impairments related to the TBI.

Summary Guidelines

1. The strategies listed in this chapter provide examples of the types of skills that can be transferred to others in a child's environment. The lists are not meant to be exhaustive; each can be developed further.

2. Each discipline that provides services for children with TBI can develop and share similar lists based on common strategies used in their profession.

3. The best way for professionals to develop such a list is to observe and self-evaluate their own work with a youngster, looking for subtle steps they take to elicit a better performance or increase the quality of a response.

4. Unless strategies such as these are recognized and shared with others with whom the child interacts, transfer of important skills will not take place. The child will be frustrated and nonsuccessful. Family members, educators, and others will feel helpless in providing adequate support.

References

Blosser, J. (1990). *Making your SLP program relevant to educational needs.* Scranton, PA: Luczerne County Schools Inservice Day.

Blosser, J., & DePompei, R. (1992). A proactive model for treating communication disorders in children and adolescents with traumatic brain injury. *Clinics in Communication Disorders, 2*(2), 52–65.

DePompei, R., & Blosser, J. (1992). *Let's organize today! A calendar of daily cognitive-communication activities for individuals with TBI.* Stow, OH: Interactive Therapeutics, Inc.

Licht, B. (1983). Cognitive-motivational factors that contribute to the achievement of learning disabled children. *Journal of Learning Disabilities, 16,* 483–490.

Reid, R., & Harris, K. R. (1993). Self-monitoring of attention versus self-monitoring of performance: Effects on attention and academic performance. *Exceptional Children, 60*(1), 29–40.

Stevens, D. D., & Englert, C. S. (1993). Making writing strategies work. *Teaching Exceptional Children, 26*(1), 34–39.

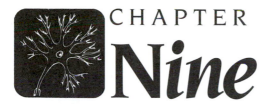

CHAPTER

Nine

Educational Issues: Planning in Advance for School Reintegration

School is the work and social place of children. Planning for functional outcomes must reflect understanding of potential challenges posed by school related issues and proactive responsiveness to those issues before they become insurmountable problems. Savage (1991) describes three key issues that are important when making initial placement decisions for children with TBI: transition between hospital and school, classification and initial placement of students, and ongoing educational programming. According to Savage, the initial transition from a biophysical environment such as the hospital to a psychodynamic school environment can create problems for the student. These problems can be mitigated if they are anticipated and confronted in advance.

At the time when educational decisions are made, additional issues arise: linking assessment activities to educational and intervention planning, fitting a child with TBI into existing educational frameworks, meeting eligibility criteria, making good class placement and service delivery decisions, selecting appropriate teaching orientations, sustaining the program and services during transitions as the child moves throughout (and then away from) the educational system, and ongoing preparation of education professionals to meet the needs of such students.

After reading this chapter, the reader will:

1. Recognize the importance of considering inclusion when planning reintegration for individuals with TBI.
2. Identify where children/adolescents with TBI fit into existing educational frameworks.
3. Learn how to conduct a classroom observation to determine the educational factors that will need to be considered when planning the school program.
4. Acknowledge the ways in which a youngster's disability affects the child's classroom performance.
5. Realize the importance of linking assessment to intervention and service delivery.
6. Suggest that team members consider teaching orientation, instructional strategies, and modifications needed in the learning environment when participating on a planning team.

Designing Treatment Programs That Promote Success

From the outset, it makes good sense to design treatment programs to promote successful inclusion of the child with TBI in school-related activities. Following is a brief description of important elements to consider when inclusion in the school environment becomes the focus of treatment:

- The student is engaged as an "active" learner versus being a passive "receiver" of information;
- Teachers coach students so they master outcomes and understand information presented versus structuring classes so students only have to memorize material and prepare for tests;
- Teachers and specialists collaborate with one another to increase a child's potential for success, sharing responsibilities and strategies;
- The physical design of the school and classroom enables children with physical disabilities as a result of TBI to have access and participate in all activities;
- The curriculum emphasizes functional learner outcomes versus textbook material. Materials that support and supplement learning are used, being adapted if necessary;

- The time spent for learning is dependent on student need versus the clock and calendar;

- Subject matter and special services are integrated into the daily classroom routine instead of separately as one subject or service at a time;

- Assessment efforts strive to determine what the child **can do** rather than **what they do not know;**

- Expectations for student performance and success is high versus related to the individual's deficits or based on the normal distribution curve;

- The school organization has flexibility so it can accommodate the student versus the student being required to fit into the system;

- Individuals and activities from the community are a part of the school rather than the school being a part of the community. (Adapted from "How does the traditional school differ from the New Ohio School?" Columbus, OH: Department of Special Education, 1993.)

Fitting Into Existing Frameworks

Public Laws 94-142, 101-476, and 102-119 all offer frameworks for providing services to children with all types of disabilities including TBI. The intent of each of these laws is to develop educational programs that are: appropriate to each youngster's individual needs, flexible enough to accommodate ongoing changes as children grow and develop, oriented toward promoting inclusion in school and community activities, focused on preparing students for the transition from school to work, and considerate of the important roles family can play. As such, educational programs that have been developed for children with disabilities other than TBI should be robust enough to meet the needs of this population. The key is in examination of existing systems and determination of how to access the best services for a given child. This makes more sense than trying to create a new "wheel." Much of the literature on TBI advises against designing classrooms exclusively for students with TBI.

When school personnel are informed that a child with TBI will be entering or returning to their school district, they need to respond proactively by identifying where this particular child fits within their current policies and procedures for serving children with special needs or disabilities. When children with TBI are reintegrated into the school setting following physical recuperation, school personnel often appear to be unprepared to discuss and meet their needs. Although they might not have encountered a child with disabilities as a result of TBI previously, they have dealt with a wide range of disabilities and children with many and varied needs.

I met with all the teachers to explain to them what TBI was like. I was looking for their help and guidance to make it a win-win situation. The communication link had to be there. (Jason's Mom)

Eligibility Criteria

Determining the appropriate school placement for a child who presents learning difficulties as a result of TBI is one of the most crucial decisions facing families and educators. To provide special services to children, school districts require documentation of the child's problems and needs. Data are gathered by considering a number of the child's traits, including social and educational characteristics, medical indicators, and qualitative performance on standardized and nonstandardized tests. Several sources of information can be used to gather data.

Observations of the child's performance in various contexts can provide two forms of information that are necessary to the decision making process: (1) additional and corroborative evidence that the student does, indeed, have a learning problem as a result of the TBI and (2) documentation of the degree to which the student's disability affects classroom performance. Observational techniques can be used to confirm the teacher's and parent's perceptions of the child's classroom behavior and performance, also providing useful diagnostic information about how a student confronts and manages the demands and expectations of the regular school program. To fulfill this purpose, the teacher and other observers who are trained to use observation as a diagnostic procedure must conduct the observations. It is helpful to have tools that can help guide the observation.

Making Class Selection and Service Delivery Decisions

Traditionally, school systems have made decisions regarding class selections, curriculum, and service provision based on predefined eligibility criteria. Eligibility criteria were originally established in accordance with federal and state eligibility rules. The practice of categorizing children by disability type has been required for documentation and states' receipt of funds. However, this system of categorizing children by their disability has sometimes worked against children, particularly those with TBI, because of the diverse nature of their impairments and needs. Current thinking in special education encourages provision of services based on a student's individual needs rather than on the category of disability exhibited. This process is referred to as noncategorical classification.

Cooley and Singer (1991) discuss four viewpoints that support non-categorical service delivery. First, the locus of academic problems experienced by children is in the environment rather than internal to the child. This means that the child's impairment must be viewed from the context in which the learning problems occur (Kameenui, 1990). This viewpoint posits that students encounter problems that may be environmentally induced. In other words, there are circumstances that exist in the environment or fall within the control of the teacher that can be managed to increase the student's potential for success. To help the student, those circumstances must be evaluated and analyzed and steps taken to make changes in the environment or people who can help need to be involved.

Second, groups of children are considered heterogeneous rather than homogeneous. A "service needs" model is followed, with placements made based on the children's learning needs rather than some artificially assigned disability label. This viewpoint is especially beneficial for children with TBI, who present such variability in their characteristics and learning needs. The third assumption is that normalization is a goal to be achieved and grouping children according to disability is detrimental rather than beneficial in achieving that goal. Rather than isolate children from school experiences and typical peers, they need to be included as much as possible.

Fourth, teaching or intervention techniques are substantially similar across categories of children. This viewpoint is very important. It supports the notion that teachers are equipped to provide good instruction. If provided with adequate support and resources and if they develop an understanding of how to select appropriate teaching techniques to meet a student's individual needs, they will be able to provide appropriate educational services. For example, instructional strategies such as teacher modeling, providing ample opportunities for student response, and guided practice are effective instructional practice regardless of a student's handicapping condition (Rosenshine, 1986).

Regardless of whether a school district adheres to a categorical or noncategorical service delivery philosophy, students' specific impairments and the effect deficits will have on learning must be documented in order to provide appropriate services. The decision regarding a child's eligibility for special education services rests with a multifactored assessment team (which must include the family). This means decisions regarding placement should be based on team judgment. The child needs to be placed in the most appropriate and least restrictive learning environment. Accommodations that are necessary to enable the child to learn in the classroom (for example, adaptations such as assistive listening devices) must be provided.

In many school districts, to qualify for services, the impairments are determined by the child's performance on standardized measures as well as through nonstandardized approaches such as structured interviews, observations, criterion-referenced and curriculum-based assessment methods. These methods can be used to confirm the reliability of the standardized measures and to determine the existence of an adverse effect on normal development, learning potential, or functioning.

To receive special education programming, related services, (physical therapy, speech-language services, occupational therapy) or even special assistance, a child's eligibility must be determined. It is often difficult to make a specific determination for children with TBI based on disability category because: the impairment conditions are not as clearly identifiable as with other populations; established evaluation protocols and instruments for this population are not available; the child may show variability in skills, appearing to have unexpected strengths and therefore not in need of services; skill areas that are mandated for evaluation to make placement decisions may not be the areas causing the greatest learning difficulty for the child; and the link between the child's problems and the effect the problem has on the child's performance within the learning setting may not be clear to those charged with making decisions about service delivery. This dilemma is not unique to children with TBI. Children with other types of disabilities, such as autism, emotional disabilities, and health-related disorders encounter the same situations. As a consequence, there has recently been a movement in education away from trying to categorize children by disability type. Currently, great gains are being made to provide individualized education and services to children based on their identified characteristics, strengths, and needs and to avoid using diagnostic labels.

Regardless of whether or not a child is "categorized" or "classified," the youngster may still be encountering difficulty in the learning situation. Failure will be inevitable unless interventions are undertaken. It may be that another service delivery method (other than special education services) will meet a child's need. Regular education personnel, such as a child's teacher or the site principal, may be appropriate individuals to coordinate intervention services.

Linking Assessment Results to Intervention

Early identification of potential learning problems and needs leads to more appropriate educational programming and service delivery. It will also result in better use of time, more meaningful placements, and improved chances for success. Assessment procedures need to be ongoing rather than conducted at specified times of the year (such as the beginning or end of a school year). All assessment activities used should be designed to provide information related to programmatic and intervention decisions. In other words, if test items and results cannot be linked to functional goals for a child, questions should be raised about the appropriateness and need for the test. Evaluators should consider the impact of environmental factors and relationships with others in the child's environment.

A number of procedures in addition to standardized testing are acceptable for describing childrens' special learning needs and gaining better insights about the child. It is very important to gain first hand information about the child from persons who are most knowledgeable about the youngster's performance, problems, strengths, and needs. This information can be gained through **structured interviews** and should include the primary caregivers as well as teachers, peers, and so on. Interviewing persons who are knowledgeable about the child can yield descriptions of aspects of a child's learning or behavior that are not available through direct assessment techniques. Examples might include self-care skills, emotional adjustment to disabilities, or problems with reestablishing friendships.

Much information can be gained by interviewing teachers who have had the opportunity to observe the child in the classroom or informal school setting. Varying the format for questioning will encourage teachers to discuss their observations and opinions about the youngster's performance. The discussion should lead to a profile of the child's cognitive-communicative skills and performance within the academic setting. In addition, recommendations for specific skills to target for treatment and strategies to use by teachers and therapists should evolve. Sample topics for discussion and interview questions that might be asked of teachers are presented in Table 9–1. This list is only presented as an example. Many other topics can be explored. Recommendations for altering the classroom environment or modifying the communication manner and style of others can be developed from the suggestions provided in Chapter 8.

Another effective technique for determining the impact of cognitive-communicative impairments on performance is to conduct **structured observations** across multiple and diverse settings and activities. This enables on-site evaluation of a child in various contexts. Through this approach, areas requiring further attention can be identified and interventions that are specific to the particular setting can be planned. Figure 9–1 illustrates the type of observation that can be carried out in the classroom setting (Holzhauser-Peters, 1988).

Table 9–1. Teacher interview.

Observation of Communication and Performance in the Classroom

Date _____   Interviewer _____

Student _____   Teacher _____

School _____   Grade _____

Instructions: Through conversations with teachers, develop a profile of the student's cognitive-communicative skills and general performance within the school setting. Highlight strengths as well as problem areas. Use the questions listed below to guide the discussion. Analyze the information gathered and use it to formulate recommendations for services.

Teacher Interview Questions

Cognitive-Communicative Skills/Performance	Target for Service?
How would you describe the student's overall performance in your class at this time? **RECOMMENDATIONS:**	
What are three successes the student has experienced recently in your classroom? **RECOMMENDATIONS:**	
Now describe three problems and talk about how you handled them. **RECOMMENDATIONS:**	
Tell me about the student's ability to tell stories, relate events, or convey information. **RECOMMENDATIONS:**	
Describe the way the student begins, ends, and maintains conversations. Is it appropriate for the situation? **RECOMMENDATIONS:**	
Explain how the student responds to humor, sarcasm, and figures of speech. **RECOMMENDATIONS:**	

Cognitive-Communicative Skills/Performance	Target for Service?
Do you feel the student recognizes and uses appropriate vocabulary considering the youngster's age and situation? **RECOMMENDATIONS:**	
Is the student's voice and intonation level appropriately matched to the situation, place, and intent? **RECOMMENDATIONS:**	
Does the student comprehend age- and grade-appropriate classroom presentations by the teacher and other students? **RECOMMENDATIONS:**	
Can the student locate details and facts to answer questions and draw conclusions? How does the youngster attempt to do so? **RECOMMENDATIONS:**	
Is the youngster able to comprehend written material from a variety of sources (newspaper, magazine, content area texts, reference materials)? Is this skill demonstrated through summarization and recall of main ideas? **RECOMMENDATIONS:**	
Describe the student's performance when following written directions to complete a task (worksheet, recipes, problems, directions for building models). **RECOMMENDATIONS:**	
Characterize the student's written work (grammar, word choice, sentence structure, organization, appearance). **RECOMMENDATIONS:**	

(continues)

Table 9-1. (continued)

Cognitive-Communicative Skills/Performance	Target for Service?
Does the student's response time permit the youngster to respond to questions when asked, participate in classroom discussions, complete assigned tasks? **RECOMMENDATIONS:**	
What motivates the student to change or improve performance efforts? **RECOMMENDATIONS:**	
Identify behaviors that might be helping this student do well. Now, identify behaviors that might be interfering with success. **RECOMMENDATIONS:**	
Based on your knowledge of children and experience in teaching, what steps do you think are necessary for helping this student at this time? **RECOMMENDATIONS:**	
What are three specific strategies you have tried to use to help this student? Why did they work or not work? **RECOMMENDATIONS:**	
PROFILE OF STUDENT'S COGNITIVE-COMMUNICATIVE AND ACADEMIC PERFORMANCE: **SUMMARY OF RECOMMENDATIONS:**	**RECOMMENDED TARGETS FOR SERVICE:**

Student's Name _____ Time of Observation _____

Classroom Teacher _____ Class Observed _____

School _____

1) Presentation of Information
   Where does teacher stand to present information?

   □ front of room _____

   □ side of room _____

   □ walks around _____

   □ Lecture _____

   □ Oral reading by various students in class _____

   □ Dittos _____

   □ Drill _____

   □ Hands-on activities _____

   □ other _____

   _____

2) Presentation of Assignments/Homework
   How are assignments presented?

   □ written on board _____

   □ verbally presented _____

   □ both _____

   □ other _____

   _____

3) Seating Arrangement
   Where is student sitting?

   □ front _____   □ back _____

   □ center of room _____   □ by window _____

   □ other _____

4) Environment—Overall
   □ Relaxed—time to do things at an even pace
   □ Fast—pushed for time

Figure 9–1. Classroom observation checklist. (Adapted from Holzhauser-Peters, L., & Huseman, D. [1988]. *Alternative service delivery models for more efficient and effective treatment programs.* Alexandria, VA: The Clinical Connection. Adapted with permission.)   (*continues*)

☐ Noise level _____

        noisy _____

        quiet _____

        moderate _____

Comments: _____

_____

5) Distractions

    ☐ Is child distracted by other children? _____

                noise _____

                other _____

    ☐ Does child distract others?

    Describe: _____

_____

6) Textbooks
Look at

        ☐ vocabulary _____

        ☐ language complexity _____

        ☐ concepts presented _____

        ☐ concepts needed to understand _____

        ☐ other _____

_____

Textbook format

        ☐ topic heads _____

        ☐ summary at end of chapter _____

        ☐ other _____

_____

7) How Does This Child Indicate What He Knows? How Does the Teacher Determine Competency Level?
Dittos

        ☐ Are dittos used a great deal?

        ☐ What skills must student possess to complete the dittos?

        ☐ Are dittos black _____

                blue _____

                clear _____

Written Essay/Papers _____

Tests
    Types of tests given
    ☐ ditto _____

    ☐ multiple choice _____

    ☐ fill in blank _____

    ☐ other _____

8) Does Student have Option of Taking Test?

    ☐ orally _____

    ☐ written _____

    ☐ both _____

9) Does the Child Participate In Class?

    ☐ Raises hand appropriately _____

    ☐ Shouts out _____

    ☐ Does child have time to respond when called upon _____
_____

    Does child respond

    ☐ immediately _____

    ☐ need more time to respond _____

    Comments: _____
_____

9) Transition
When class moves from one subject or task to another, how does teacher
cue children into transition?

    ☐ physically (with body movements) _____

    ☐ verbally _____

    ☐ bell _____

    ☐ other _____

    ☐ Does student pick up on this cue? _____

10) Child's Organizational Skills
Does child remember?

    ☐ homework assignments _____

    ☐ books needed to take home _____

    ☐ what books and materials to take to next class _____

Figure 9–1. (*continues*)

☐ schedule of classes and daily events

Comments: _____

_____

11) Study Skills
Does the child know how to study?

☐ to remember only important information _____

☐ scan chapter first to review headings _____

☐ read chapter summary first _____

☐ get clues by looking at ditto first to determine how to do and the read directions _____

☐ how to take notes _____

☐ how to outline _____

Comments _____

_____

12) Verbal Organizational Skills

Student:

☐ answers simple questions requiring a one word or 1–2 sentence response

☐ relates information in an understandable cohesive manner

☐ during conversations with adults

☐ during conversations with friends

☐ during class discussions through

written assignments _____

oral presentations _____

☐ communicates wants and needs

☐ relates the sequence of events in the proper order

☐ communicates something that has happened recently _____

in the distant past _____

will happen in the future _____

☐ relates feelings

☐ relates thoughts

☐ relates opinions

Comments: _____

_____

13) Requests For Assistance
When the student has difficulty with a task he

☐ requests assistance   ☐ gives up   ☐ other (Describe) _____

_____

14) General

Does the child seem to exhibit skills comparable to other children in the class or does the student stand out? Describe how the student "stands out" from the group. Give examples of specific situations when the student "stands out" and also when he "fits in."

_____
_____
_____
_____

Figure 9–1. (*continued*)

The educational curriculum represents a series of skills or behaviors children must master. When a child demonstrates difficulty performing learning tasks, there is an indication that intervention and support are needed. Therefore, **curriculum-based assessment** approaches can provide a useful format for exploring children's special learning needs and linking assessment, the curriculum, and intervention (Bagnato, Neisworth, & Capone, 1986; Dellegrotto, 1993). In curriculum-based assessment, the material to be learned is used as the basis for assessing the degree to which it has been learned (Tucker, 1985). The student's performance is measured in reference to the curriculum rather than standardized tests. It is a good procedure for determining the instructional needs of a student based on the student's ongoing performance within existing course content (Gickling & Havertape, 1981). This approach can be particularly appropriate in working with children with TBI because it provides a system for ongoing assessment in terms of expected outcomes. It is useful at two different times. First, prior to making a grade or class placement recommendation, the curriculum for that placement should be thoroughly reviewed to determine the skills a child would need to be able to demonstrate to be successful. Secondly, when a child hits a "snag" because of expected rate or quality of performance, modifications in teaching strategies should be made. The tools needed for conducting curriculum-based assessments are the printed curriculum with clearly identified materials and student goals (Bigge, 1988).

A similar assessment method educators find useful is **criterion-refer-enced assessment**. In this approach, the child's performance in a specific skill area is described. The child's performance is not compared to or ranked in relation to other students, but, instead, is described by mastery achieved in a given area.

Portfolio assessment can provide good opportunities for assessing a child's performance. For this method, a collection of the child's work is gathered. Review helps planners gain a good understanding of the child's efforts, progress, and achievements in various subject areas. Professionals who support the use of this evaluative technique encourage soliciting the child's input to select the materials that best represent the individual's performance.

Programs for children with other types of disabilities require evaluation of performance on at least an annual basis. Because children with TBI show changes over time, more frequent reviews of their performance are necessary. In lieu of formalized testing, some of the alternative assessment procedures presented above can be used. If teachers are involved in assessment procedures, they will become more adept at recognizing changes in a child.

Teaching Orientation

One of the most critical educational decisions to be made is selection of the teaching orientation that will most help a child. The planning team needs to decide if a child will benefit more from an orientation that emphasizes "process" or "product." In a process orientation, the instructional activities and strategies are geared toward helping the child understand the "how to do's of learning." In a product orientation, the focus is on completion of specified instructional tasks, such as writing an essay, completing a required number of math problems, or finishing a requisite number of workbook pages. Some refer to these as cognitive/learning strategy intervention approaches (Brown & Palincsar, 1982; Ryan, Short, & Weed, 1986; Wong, Perry, & Sawatsky, 1986). Because of the resulting deficits and characteristics associated with TBI, it is reasonable to expect that children with TBI can benefit from the use of a process-oriented approach.

Combining a process/product orientation may actually yield the most functional results. This can be accomplished by simultaneously centering teaching on completion of products (class and homework assignments), while helping the student understand the strategy needed for successful completion (maintaining attention, identifying important facts and topics, organizational skills). A combined effort helps the student best meet educational expectations. When this instructional model is used, the student's overall performance is improved and there is a higher level of task engagement. For example, instead of being concerned about the number of pages to be completed or length of an essay, the focus is on the demands of a particular task and skills necessary for successful completion.

When recommendations to use a particular teaching orientation are made to some teachers (especially general educators), they may resist. This may be because they were not trained to make individualized adaptations to student's needs during their professional training. They may feel incompetent to do so and might resist the placement of a child with such needs in their classroom. Teachers may also feel that individualizing instruction will compromise the educational needs of other students in class. Some teachers automatically use a combined approach; others will be willing to try if provided with assistance and suggestions. Placements with such teachers and those who are willing to try a combined approach should be sought. Some classrooms (such as special education settings) incorporate a process orientation in the curriculum. Special education teachers are secure in the process of individualizing work. They know how to analyze learning tasks, adapt curricula, and measure student progress. Often this is why placement into special education classes is the recommended service delivery model. A child can even do well in a class placement that emphasizes a product orientation if support is given through tutoring or special services. All of this suggests the need to collaborate when reintegrating a child into the school setting. In schools with an intervention assistance team model, teachers and specialists can provide the needed support to one another. Graden (1989) recommends the use of teacher-teacher problem solving, teacher-special services problem solving, and prescribed use of teacher problem solving as essential when trying to develop effective programming to meet the complex needs of students who experience difficulty in the school setting.

Selecting Appropriate Instructional Strategies

Educating children with TBI requires sensitivity to the behavioral and learning problems these students present. Most teachers are interested in helping a child with TBI reintegrate and successfully achieve in the school setting. Teachers need to know that there are numerous instructional strategies they can use to provide support and assistance. It is important to help teachers understand that most of the strategies they need for working with children with TBI are already in their "bag of teaching tricks." They need simply to learn to recognize which strategies need to be applied in response to specific situations and problems that arise. They need to be given ideas and suggestions for arranging the teaching and learning environment to enhance a child's potential. Finally, they need recommendations for adapting and altering the curriculum and instructional requirements to meet a child's needs.

All of this suggests that the extent and impact of problems a child experiences in the educational setting can be reduced if the educational approach used is more individualized and tailored to meet unique needs. Teachers can evoke a more positive experience with a child with TBI if they strive to create a learning environment that is more conducive to the student's needs and selectively apply a variety of teaching strategies and techniques. The literature in developmental psychology, special education, communicative disorders, and education can lead us to greater understanding of the types of instructional strategies that can be useful with this group of children. Rowjewski (1991) suggests six general approaches to teaching that have been successful for students with disabilities: (1) individualization of instructional techniques and evaluation based on individual student ability, (2) flexibility in teaching and evaluation methods, (3) collaboration with special education and support staff, (4) use of prestated objectives or competencies, (5) multiple evaluation methods, and (6) emphasis on positive aspects of student performance.

The team must also make decisions about performance criteria. It is not unusual to use alternative or modified grading approaches with children who exhibit disabilities. If, indeed, learning rather than task completion is the goal of education, then there should be flexibility in the grading system used. Students can be provided with an opportunity to retake tests, if a grade achieved independently is below expectation or failing. The administration of the second test can be modified to provide supports such as restructuring the administration procedures (reading the test to the child) or modifying the mode of response to test questions (having verbal answers instead of written). The second test score can stand alone or be averaged with the first. Another alternative sometimes used is to raise the mark by one level, if the child's performance is independent and if effort was demonstrated. There should be an indication on the child's report card indicating that grade modifications were made.

Modifying the Learning Environment

As discussed earlier, the climate and structure of the learning environment can directly influence students' performance, behavior, and learning. Once the expectations and demands of the learning environment are identified, recommendations should be made for modifying or structuring the environment to support the student and increase learning potential (Solomon, Schaps, Watson, & Battistich, 1992). The ideal learning environment should be structured to encourage learning, provide opportunities for student-to-student and student-to-teacher interactions, and compensate for learning deficiencies. This implies flexibility, diversity, and functionality.

Gloeckler and Simpson (1988) discuss how three features of the educational environment interact with one another to affect the learning potential for children with disabilities. Those features are the psychological environment, the social environment, and the physical environment.

The teacher sets the scene for the psychological environment. A positive learning atmosphere is created by accepting students as individuals; relaying expectations in a clear and concise way; responding appropriately, fairly, and consistently to students' needs and behaviors; and skillfully engaging students in learning tasks and classroom activities. The teacher's attitude when children experience problems and the approach used for teaching difficult material set the tone for the psychological environment. When selecting a class placement for a youngster with TBI, it is important to seek out those teachers that create a positive psychological learning environment.

A second feature, the social environment, is a particularly important consideration for children with TBI. Social relationships and interactions are often affected as a result of cognitive-communicative impairments. Friendships may be difficult to renew, establish, or maintain. Classrooms that promote group activity, peer interactions, and sharing foster development of these skills in youngsters who are having difficulty.

The physical environment needs to be assessed to determine if any barriers will interfere with learning. These might include physical, auditory, or visual interferences. Plans should be made to eliminate or modify barriers and decrease distractions. Children with TBI function better in environments with a sense of order. Often this can be created by structuring and manipulating the physical environment of the classroom to facilitate organization. Teachers can use strategies such as posting due dates and schedules in visible places, presenting directions in a simple manner, and clearly identifying the location of learning materials. The child's physical location in the room may need to be modified to permit better attention to the teacher as well as learning tasks and materials. There should be ease of movement around the classroom and throughout the building, especially for youngsters who have physical disabilities as a result of their TBI. Devices promoting better efficiency and accuracy should be encouraged. These can include calculators, word processors, tape recorders, computers, and so on.

During planning meetings, numerous aspects of the learning environment should be discussed and modified to create the most appropriate climate for the student with TBI: degree of structure; daily routine; requirements for participation; adaptations needed to facilitate inclusion and participation; learning space and materials; time allocation for completion of assignments; and necessary alterations or modifications in grading practices. These variables will vary from child to child, classroom to classroom, and teacher to teacher. Yet, it is variables such as these that will lead to difficulty on school return or as the child moves through the numerous transitions through school. Each of these issues should be discussed thoroughly when planning the first reintegration into the school setting following physical recuperation from the TBI as well as before each subsequent transition as the student moves through the educational setting and into the work setting.

Sustaining Programs and Service Delivery Through Transitions

As children transition through various contexts and situations, there is a real danger that programming will be interrupted. Steps must be taken to ensure that this does not happen. This can be accomplished by establishing liaisons to pass along valuable information about the child's needs and treatment strategies each time a child makes a new transition. The best course of action is to teach family members as much as possible about their child and his or her needs. Then, they can be liaisons to facilitate relationships between professionals from one facility to another.

Summary Guidelines

1. Because school is the work and social center for children and adolescents, it is reasonable to consider important aspects of the educational setting when planning and implementing treatment.

2. Treatment programs should strive to promote inclusion of the individual with TBI within avenues and activities that exist for individuals who do not have disabilities.

3. The frameworks within the school setting that exist for children and adolescents with other types of disabilities are robust enough to accommodate the needs of youngsters with TBI; but, professionals

and family must come to understand this and utilize the best resources available.

4. Class selection and service delivery decisions should be based on the behaviors and characteristics (strengths as well as needs) demonstrated by the child/adolescent.

5. A broad range of assessment techniques are available to help professionals and families make sound decisions regarding treatment needs.

6. Thought should be given to the teaching orientation, instructional strategies, and learning environment selected for youth with TBI.

7. We need to take steps to ensure that there is careful planning to be sure that treatment and intervention efforts are continuous as an individual transitions from one situation to the next.

References

Bagnato, S. J., Neisworth, J. T., & Capone, A. (1986). Curriculum-based assessment for the young exceptional child: Rationale and review. *Topics in Early Childhood Special Education, 6*(2), 97–110.

Bigge, J. (1988). *Curriculum based assessment for special education students.* Mountain View, CA: Mayfield Publishing Co.

Brown, A. L., & Palincsar, A. S. (1982). Inducing strategic learning from texts by means of informed self-control training. *Topics in Learning and Learning Disabilities, 2,* 1–17.

Cooley, E., & Singer, G. (1991). On serving students with head injury: Are we reinventing a wheel that doesn't roll? In R. DePompei & J. Blosser (Eds.), School reentry following head injury [Special issue]. *Journal of Head Trauma Rehabilitation, 6*(1), 47–55.

Dellegrotto, J. (1993). *Curriculum-based assessment concepts for the speech and language clinician.* Summerdale, PA: Capital Area School District Intermediate Unit.

Gickling, E., & Havertape, J. (1981). *Curriculum-based assessment.* Minneapolis: University of Minnesota.

Gloeckler, T., & Simpson, C. (1988). *Exceptional students in regular classrooms: Challenges, services, and methods.* Mountain View, CA: Mayfield Publishing Company.

Graden, J. L. (1989). Redefining "prereferal" intervention as intervention assistance: Collaboration between general and special education. *Exceptional Children, 56*(3), 227–231.

Holzhauser-Peters, L., & Husemann, D. A. (1988). *Alternative service delivery models for more efficient and effective treatment programs.* Alexandria, VA: The Clinical Connection.

Kameenui, E. J., & Simmons, D. C. (1990). *Designing instructional strategies: The prevention of academic learning problems.* Columbus, OH: Merrill Publishing.

Rojewski, J. W. (1992). Grading secondary vocational education students with disabilities. *Exceptional Children, 59*(1), 68–76.

Rosenshine, B. (1986). Synthesis of research on explicit teaching. *Educational Leadership, 43*(7), 60–69.

Ryan, E. B., Short, E., & Weed, K. A. (1986). The role of cognitive strategy training in improving the academic performance of learning disabled children. *Journal of Learning Disabilities, 19*, 521–529.

Savage, R. (1991). Identification, classification, and placement issues for students with traumatic brain injuries. In R. DePompei & J. Blosser (Eds.), School reentry following head injury [Special issue]. *The Journal of Head Trauma Rehabilitation, 6*(1), 1–9.

Solomon, D., Schaps, E., Watson, M., & Battistich, V. (1992). Creating caring school and classroom communities for all students. In R. A. Villa, J. S. Thousand, W. Stainback, & S. Stainback (Eds.), *Restructuring for caring and effective education.* Baltimore: Paul H. Brookes Publishing Company.

Tucker, J. (1985). Curriculum-based assessment: An introduction. *Exceptional Children, 52*, 199–204.

Wong, B. Y. L., Wong, R., Perry, N., & Sawatsky, D. (1986). The efficacy of self questioning, summarization strategy for use by underachievers and learning disabled adolescents in social studies. *Learning Disabilities Focus, 2*, 20–31.

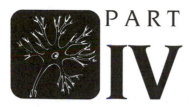

Application of a Proactive Approach to Treatment of a Youngster With TBI

*Months later I watch people in
"intensive care" on TV. Tears flow
as memories of my brother's hospital
stay come flooding back.
I go over and hug him and thank God he survived.
Then my attention returns to the TV and I feel betrayed.
This person opens his eyes and is perfectly normal.
There is no waiting or questioning or deficits or things
that gradually come back.
In one scene this person is almost dead and the next scene
he is out running around and is perfectly normal.
Is it any surprise then that I had no idea how long the
recovery process would take or what it would consist of?*

Linda Offenhartz (1994)
Personal Journal maintained during
her brother's experiences with TBI

One of the most difficult challenges for service providers and families is to develop a plan over time that will help the child/adolescent with TBI throughout the remainder of his/her life. Families often do not understand the duration of the learning and social problems that may exist.

Professionals and family members of children/adolescents who experience problems after a traumatic brain injury need information to help them understand the youngster's disabilities and how to provide help when needed. Knowledge about how to conduct assessments is critical to helping youth to reintegrate into home, school, work, and community. Ability to provide outcome-based, functional intervention is essential to persons helping youth so they can be successful in those environments. However, it is the appropriate application of all information obtained and the collaboration of everyone involved that is most essential to the reintegration process.

Part IV outlines an integrated, proactive approach to intervention for a child who sustained a TBI. Because the primary workplace of children is the school, the information presented focuses on reintegrating the child, Alan, to that setting. Based on the examples provided, the reader should be able to generalize the recommendations to other settings.

The reader should learn to:

1. Recognize the importance of coordinating communication about the youngster between professionals and family and among professionals within and between agencies.

2. Understand the need to obtain current information about the qualifications for entrance to referral facilities, such as requirements for special education placements, provisions for referral to work-study programs, etc.

3. Describe the need for linking assessment results to intervention that is appropriate to functioning in the environments that are important to the child/adolescent.

4. Apply modifications of the environment or persons in the environment to the specific needs of the youngster.

5. Advocate for ongoing transitions throughout the youngster's life.

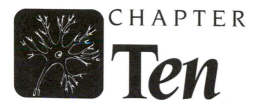

CHAPTER

Ten

Applying Proactive Planning and Intervention

A Case Study

Alan, age 14, was driving a 4-wheel recreational vehicle when he tumbled into a culvert. He was found unconscious hours after the accident. He was airlifted to a regional children's hospital. The CT scan identified a depressed skull fracture, cerebral contusions, and an intercerebral hemorrhage in the left parieto-temporal areas. The skull fracture was elevated and debridement completed. Estimated Glasgow Coma Scale (GSC) was 9. There was no elevated intracranial pressure or seizure. Two days later, GSC was 11. Repeat neuroradiological procedures identified some focal edema and sequelae of the hemorrhage. EEGs showed marked diffuse slowing in the left parietotemporal area. Alan also demonstrated a significant flat conductive hearing loss of 59dB in the left ear.

Within 2 weeks, Alan's GCS was at 13. He ambulated with assistance, demonstrated poor fine motor control, and exhibited no expressive speech. Cognitive deficits were obvious. He was on a regular diet. He was referred to a residential rehabilitation facility for continuation of all rehabilitation services. He remained in the rehabilitation facility for 6 weeks before being sent home.

At the time of discharge from the rehabilitation facility, recommendations were made for continuation of rehabilitation services (speech-language, and occupational therapy) by staff at a local hospital and then reintegration to school when his school reopened after summer recess (about 5 weeks). The family was advised to contact the school immediately to alert them to the Alan's special needs upon returning to school. Written copies of the rehabilitation facility's evaluations and recommendations were made immediately available to the hospital and school staff. One phone conversation between the school psychologist and rehabilitation facility psychologist took place at the time of discharge. General suggestions for teaching students with TBI were provided.

Following are several brief excerpts from the rehabilitation facility's discharge report and recommendations.

Family History

Alan is the second of three children. At the time of his TBI, he lived with his parents, Jim (age 44) and JoAnn (age 40) and his younger brother Michael (age 12). His sister Nancy was a college freshman and lived away from home. The mother was supportive and interested in helping Alan in any way possible. The father has expressed concern and willingness to help but had little direct involvement during Alan's stay in the rehabilitation facility.

Alan's birth was normal according to his mother. He was born at full term. All developmental milestones were reached at the expected time periods. He had no history of major illnesses or hospitalizations. He was described as a friendly, outgoing child during his preschool years. He reportedly did not like to watch TV or play quiet games. He preferred playing outside with one or two friends. He is right handed. He got along well with his siblings and enjoyed golfing with his father.

Educational History

Alan had progressed through school in regular class placements through seventh grade (just completed at the time of the accident). The most recent report card prior to the accident indicated that he received credit for all seventh grade classes. He obtained a "D" in physical science, "Cs" in English and American history, and "Bs" in math, reading, and physical education. He received tutoring for reading during the school day from third through seventh grades. His last reading test (prior to the injury) placed him at a sixth grade reading level. He told his teachers and parents that he didn't like reading or math. Teachers considered him to be cooperative, outgoing, pleasant, and easy to get along with in the classroom. Alan preferred team sports over individual sports.

Test Results at the Time of Discharge

Prior to discharge, staff made attempts to administer several formal tests including the PPVT (*Peabody Picture Vocabulary Test*), the CELF-R (*Clinical Evaluation of Functional Language-Revised*), the *Boston Naming Test*, and the *Woodcock-Johnson Psychoeducational Test Battery*. Only the PPVT was completely administered. Alan obtained an age equivalency score of 9–6. Observations of several skill and behavioral areas were made during informal activities and testing and revealed the following information.

Attention

Alan exhibited a visual attention span of about 1 minute. He responded by pointing to pictures and matched objects and pictures. He had difficulty matching pictures to short descriptive sentences. When asked to cancel out numbers or similar words, he took 2–4 times longer than is normally expected. He was able to visually track up and down the page, looking for matches (right to left progression is more common). He could watch a video or TV program for about 10 minutes and then became distracted. His auditory attention span was dependent on the topics presented, with family and sports receiving the most careful attention. He was unable to respond to sentences of more than 4 to 7 words and directions for testing were difficult for him.

Language

Expressive communication was limited to single words that were expressed with long pauses and some vocalized struggle for productions. Alan was able to name seven of the pictures on the *Boston Naming Test*. Naming was completed with processing time that was 3–4 times longer than expected. Familiar nouns and phrases were spontaneously emerging during conversations. Speech requiring formulation of ideas in phrases rather than more automatic responses was only beginning to be initiated. Formalized testing was unsuccessful at the time of discharge from the rehabilitation facility.

Some questions were raised about receptive language skills. Alan often misunderstood directions and seemingly did not understand what was being requested of him during the testing. He responded better when given multiple-choice response formats. The hearing loss was acknowledged as contributing to the lack of auditory responsiveness. Treatment was initiated for the misarticulated ossicular chain and an assistive listening device was employed for the left ear during evaluation and treatment sessions. Differentiation of central auditory processing problems versus dysnomia continued to cause difficulty for the staff. When he was at the rehabilitation facility, the dysnomia appeared to be the primary area of difficulty and receptive language skills appeared to be intact as long as it could be confirmed that he was hearing the message.

It was difficult to form conclusions about Alan's pragmatic language skills, because verbalizations were limited. Observations during therapy-related activities showed that Alan was able to initiate communication through a series of vocalizations and single words. His actions were impulsive, distractible, and somewhat disinhibited. Although he was compliant and cooperative, he was not motivated to do school-related activities and was withdrawn. He did not engage in social activities with other patients at the facility. He showed minimal awareness of his problems. When reminded of the difficulties he experienced, he acted surprised.

Motor Skills

Gross motor skills were appropriate. Fine motor skills were slow and awkward, but not markedly impaired relative to the general population or casual observer. Speed and efficiency of fine motor skills were observably affected.

Reasoning

Alan was able to complete quantitative reasoning that depended on counting and matching visually. He was unable to demonstrate any verbal reasoning, probably due to limited verbal output abilities.

Executive Functioning

Alan showed marked difficulties with concept formation and retention, attentional abilities, and related executive abilities. The organizational and language components were so involved that no formal assessments were completed.

Summary and Recommendations Made by Staff of the Rehabilitation Facility at Discharge

Testing and observations indicated that Alan had significant cognitive-communicative dysfunctions and that there was diffuse brain damage causing the dysfunctioning. Functioning levels in all tests attempted to place him at the lowest levels or could not be interpreted because of lack of responsiveness to testing. Staff indicated that they anticipated that much improvement would occur within the next few months, particularly with expressive and receptive language skills, confusion, and fine motor skills. No attempt was made to estimate the extent of improvement that might occur. Specific recommendations were:

1. Outpatient therapy to include speech-language therapy, occupational therapy, counseling for Alan, family, and close friends.

2. Evaluation by school personnel to determine appropriate placement for school in the Fall. Suggestions included placement in a structured, self-contained classroom with a minimum number of students. The optimal class atmosphere would be relatively quiet and free of auditory and visual distractions. Placement with children who exhibited emotional or behavioral disabilities was not recommended. Related services of speech-language therapy and occupational therapy within the school day would be initiated. Because Alan experienced some problems with memory and had difficulty finding his way to various locations within the rehabilitation facility, it was recommended that assistance be provided for daily orientation, maintaining his class schedule, and moving from place to place in the school building.

3. Reevaluation periodically (every 6 to 8 weeks) to monitor progress and detect changes needed in scheduling and programming was set.

4. Maintenance of close contact among parents, school personnel, and rehabilitation staff. Encouragement of individuals who are working with Alan most closely to maintain a log of activities, problems, and questions.

5. Monitoring of emotional and behavioral performance during the next school year. If significant problems arise, refer immediately for psychological and guidance services.

6. Begin to develop a transitional plan for future education or employment to ensure appropriate academic placement.

The above report is meant to merely exemplify the type of information and recommendations often sent when a youngster is discharged from one facility to the next. More comprehensive information and materials would likely be available and exchanged; however, it is not possible to include everything here. **It is important to realize that it is this foundation on which future planning must be based. Someone has to ensure that the recommendations will be effectively carried out.** The remainder of this chapter covers how to apply proactive planning and treatment processes for planning Alan's return to school.

Proactive Responses

Proactive Response 1

Make sure everyone who will be closely involved with the youngster develops a complete understanding of the nature and scope of the traumatic brain injury and how it is likely to affect performance of social, school, and work activities.

Characteristics and terminology associated with Alan's TBI and treatment should be clearly and concisely explained to all members of his family periodically as he progresses from stage to stage during his stay in the medical facility, when he goes to the rehabilitation facility, and after he leaves for outpatient treatment and return to school. Other important individuals, such as teachers, friends, and relatives should be "brought into the information loop" as early as possible to promote understanding of what Alan and his family are going through and what is ahead of them. The family should be encouraged to assign one family member as the "notetaker." A log of progress and answers to questions given by various staff members can be recorded for later reference and to assist others in understanding what has happened to Alan. Family members should be provided with materials (written, audio, and video) about TBI and services for individuals with TBI to help them increase their knowledge base.

Proactive Response 2

Adopt a proactive philosophy of service delivery.

Clinical decision making and modes of service delivery evolve from the knowledge and competency of the professionals who are delivering the services. Because of the nature and extent of Alan's disabilities as a result of his injury, it will be inevitable for numerous professionals representing a variety of philosophical orientations to be involved in planning and implementing his treatment. This can cause programming to be disjointed and confusing to the family. It would be wise for the practitioners involved in Alan's programs to examine their own philosophies and discuss those of others. Consensus and coordination among practitioners about future program design and directions will strengthen the efforts of all who are involved. It will also help create a pathway for the participation of others in future programming for Alan.

Proactive Response 3

Form a dynamic, interactive, coordinated team for planning and implementing services and schooling.

To maintain consistency and keep treatment forward moving, it would be in Alan's and his family's best interests to form a dynamic, interactive, coordinated team with a shared philosophy, mission, goals, and objectives. Together, the team can analyze Alan's needs, predict challenges, and formulate creative solutions. As transitions occur throughout Alan's growth and development, the composition of the team will necessarily change. It would be most ideal if Alan's family could learn to function as team leaders, because they will be responsible for coordinating the team efforts and Alan's transitions for years to come. Practitioners should encourage as high a level of family involvement as possible given the family's interests and capabilities. At various points in Alan's programming (at the rehabilitation facility, at the local hospital, and in the school setting) an individualized family/peer intervention plan (IF/PIP) should be created to confirm the information the family and others need to obtain at a given time and how delivery of the information will be accomplished.

Proactive Response 4

Form intra- and interagency networks and initiate collaborative training and development projects.

As Alan moves from program to program, services may become disconnected and fragmented. To avoid this common problem, it would be wise for professionals at each setting to make contact with one another before, during, and prior to dismissal from each particular setting. It doesn't matter who initiates the contact first as long as it is initiated by someone. Ideally, a team composed of Alan's family, a school representative, and a staff member from the local hospital should meet (in person or through a conference call) to begin to form a working network. Given the time frame in Alan's situation, the rehab team should probably contact professionals at the local hospital and school system. Each should make a point to exchange information about their program, services offered, goals established for Alan, methods that have been successful and the like. As individuals are encountered who do not understand TBI or are unaware of techniques for managing youngsters with TBI, professional training and development should be undertaken. The modes to be used for presentation of information will likely vary. For example, Alan's older sister may need to gain information through written materials and audiotapes because she lives away from home. The teachers he will have when he returns to school can be provided information during an intervention assistance team meeting or at the time the individualized education program (IEP) or individualized family service plan (IFSP) is established. Oftentimes, school districts offer in-service days for teachers prior to the beginning of school. Perhaps Alan's teachers can be encouraged to attend an in-service meeting on the topic of TBI or spend a portion of the day meeting with staff from the rehabilitation center or hospital.

Proactive Response 5

Devise a comprehensive assessment protocol that considers three major aspects: the impairments resulting from the TBI as well as strengths, the demands and expectations of the situations to be encountered, and the responsibilities and contributions of others. (This assessment protocol should be repeated periodically as the youngster's skills improve and as new situations are encountered.)

On discharge from the rehabilitation facility, Alan will enter a very complex and dynamic world. The quality of his performance will depend on many factors. His performance is likely to vary with the situations he encounters. The fact that his expressive language skills are impaired will most likely cause him and those around him great difficulty. A comprehensive profile of his communication skills should be developed including the problems he has and the way he attempts to communicate. An analysis should be conducted of the environmental situations in which verbal communication is necessary in order for Alan to communicate his basic wants, needs, and frustrations. The persons who he will encounter will carry the burden of interpreting his communication attempts and responding accordingly. Their capability to do so and the steps needed to increase their competency should be evaluated.

Proactive Response 6

Analyze the situations the individual will encounter and develop appropriate transition (and education) plans.

The transition plan developed should have multiple facets. Most importantly, it should address Alan's immediate discharge from the rehabilitation facility, services at the local hospital, return to school (including the work he will need to do to get ready), placement issues, teaching techniques, and specified times for reevaluation and revision of the plan. Because Alan is a teenager, he should be included in discussions about his problems, the services he receives, and future plans. His thoughts, opinions, and feelings should be sought and incorporated into the plan. Vocational preparation should be a topic for exploration. Determine steps each person should take to effectively assist Alan and the skills the helpers will need for success. Attempt to reintroduce Alan to the activities he engaged in prior to the injury. Anticipate problems and think about solutions. In Alan's case, he will need a method for communicating his needs until his verbal communication skills improve. He will need to rebuild friendships. Friends will expect him to be the outgoing person he was prior to the accident. They will need help in understanding the changes in him and learning to accept the differences and participate in the recovery process. He will need to be supported while adjusting to a new type of class placement.

Proactive Response 7

Continually scan and analyze to determine the problems and situation that lie ahead for the individual. Revise the transition plan accordingly.

Alan made great strides in his physical recovery from the time of his injury to the point where he was discharged from the rehabilitation and ready to receive services on an out-patient basis. Rehab personnel anticipated that he would continue to make positive changes. Select a class placement that will accommodate his needs at entry, but be prepared to make a quick change as skills improve. Work with teachers to help them understand the techniques in their teaching repertoire that will benefit Alan most. It is expected that his expressive language skills will improve enough for him to communicate a message and for people to understand him. There may even be a tendency for some to think he is "doing okay" once he begins to "sound okay." Caution is recommended at this point. Someone who is aware of the problems and ramifications often associated with TBI will have to keep others alert so Alan doesn't fall between the cracks. It would be ideal if the someone could be Alan's parents and the school personnel because they will have the best opportunities to observe Alan on a daily basis and as he changes over time. Continue to keep others informed about Alan and to refine their skills so they can be effective participants in Alan's efforts to achieve a good quality of life.

School Reintegration Planning Guide

Following steps such as those listed throughout this book and on The School Reintegration Planning Guide (Figure 10–1) will promote a smooth transition from the medical or rehabilitation environment to the school setting. The Planning Guide is designed to be used by school personnel, family members, rehabilitation and/or medical staff. The purpose is to get people talking and working together to learn more about the student's strengths and needs, to discuss potential challenges for the student, and to propose solutions to problems before they occur.

ACTION TO BE TAKEN	PERSON/S RESPONSIBLE	DATE
I. PRIOR TO RETURNING TO SCHOOL		
A. Identify one individual at each facility who will serve as liaison and coordinator of networking. (Make the decision jointly with family.)		
B. Follow all established school policies and procedures for exchanging information and communicating with other agencies.		
C. Schedule a meeting to discuss plans for the student. Invite family members and people who have been involved with the student's rehabilitation as well as former and new educators.		
D. Compile as much information about the student as possible based on comments from family and friends, test data, and observations.		
E. Establish a plan for exchanging information, educating one another, and developing an effective reintegration plan.		
F. Learn about the student's present status (including impairments, strengths, needs, interests).		
1. Obtain medical/rehabilitation records.		
2. Find out about the medical aspects of the injury (nature and extent of damage).		
3. Construct a record of treatment history and progress.		
4. Generate a profile characterizing the student's skills and capabilities as well as needs at the time of reintegration. Be prepared to update frequently as changes occur.		
5. Identify the physical, cognitive-communicative, and social behaviors that are likely to interfere with learning and social activities at school.		
6. Obtain samples of the student's work that are representative of current capabilities and levels of performance.		
G. Relate information gained to the general requisite needs for educational success.		

Figure 10–1. The school reintegration planning guide.

1. Discuss characteristics of the school and various class settings, expectations for performance, routines, learning materials, classmates, and so on.		
2. Determine the student's readiness to participate in school activities based on the recognized demands of the educational setting.		
3. Discuss options and educational choices available to the student. Strive for a high level of inclusion.		
H. Evaluate the school's readiness and capabilities for meeting the student's needs at the time.		
1. Discuss applicable school policies and procedures regarding meeting a student's special needs (including special education and related service options, eligibility criteria, staff capabilities, and so on.)		
2. Make arrangements for pertinent assessments to obtain information for educational planning.		
3. Determine obstacles that may interfere with successful reintegration. Look at the student critically from the perspective of program offerings, personnel, and so on.		
4. Search for the most appropriate class selection and personnel.		
5. Determine how to modify, eliminate, or reduce the obstacles. Establish objectives (for the environment, the educators, the student).		
I. Search for the most appropriate class and personnel to meet the student's needs. Consider several critical elements:		
1. Review the instructional objectives associated with the selected class.		
2. Determine if the objectives are compatible with the student's capabilities and long-term needs.		
3. Analyze the socialization characteristics, demands, and needs.		

(continues)

4. Observe the classroom climate and environment.		
5. Evaluate the teacher's willingness to learn and/or level of understanding of youngsters with TBI.		
6. Determine if key educator characteristics are present including: flexibility, acceptance, patience, positive, supportive attitude, competence, and repertoire of teaching techniques.		
J. Prepare an Individualized Education Plan (IEP) addressing the student's needs and confirming specific recommendations for modification of the environment and techniques educators and others can use to help the student.		
II. AFTER THE REINTEGRATION		
A. Maintain ongoing communication about the student's performance through an organized flow of information.		
B. Look ahead to the next stages in the student's educational experience. Determine other educators who will be involved. Formulate a plan for preparing them to meet the student's needs.		
C. Develop peer support systems by: educating peers, alerting them to the student's problems and ways for helping, and providing opportunities for involvement in extracurricular activities.		
D. Gather family and personnel who have been involved with the student. Summarize the student's performance and the overall success of the reintegration. Discuss satisfaction with learner outcomes.		
E. Decide what program aspects can be changed, eliminated, or increased to raise future potential.		
F. Prepare a transition plan to enable proactive response to situations to be encountered.		
G. Additional Items of Importance		

Figure 10-1. (continued)

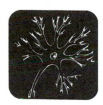

Epilogue: Down the Yellow Brick Road

Our Dorothy travels a long and twisting yellow brick road. Her friends search for many of the characteristics that she herself needs—a new brain, a heart, and courage. Sometimes, we as clinicians believe that the journey is too hard, the problems too complex, the witches too real. We are sure that we are not Merlin or the Wizard and we have few answers. It is during those times that we need to revisit the Wizard, himself. He really wasn't such a genius you know! But he did know how to collaborate, dispense encouragement, and employ proven techniques to help those around him. He also wasn't afraid to try a new idea or create another challenge.

Proactive planning is our wizardry. Considering all communication environments and partners in those environments is a means of providing travel markers along the yellow brick road. Knowing that assessment and treatment are interrelated and must be thoroughly developed on an individual basis is a way to encourage Dorothy when she falters. Recognizing the support Dorothy's peers, the Scarecrow, Cowardly Lion, and Tin Man, provided, encourages us to involve family and peers more consistently. It is possible to help Dorothy to develop compensatory strategies and to believe in herself so that she can melt the witches away. We can be the Wizard. We can anticipate problems and offer proactive solutions. We possess the knowledge and skills to help Dorothy along that road and we can help Dorothy to click the heels of those slippers and return home!

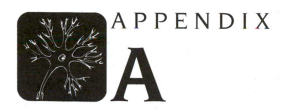

Professional Training and Development: Targeting Necessary Competencies

Identification of the nature of TBI

- Target competencies
  - Educators will have a common base of understanding of the nature of TBI and related medical aspects from which to discuss implications for the educational setting
- Objectives
  - to increase awareness of the causes, incidence, and significance of TBI
  - to understand the demographic, medical, and recovery aspects; ranges of disability; and resulting deficits
- Topics for discussion
  - causes, incidence, pathophysiology, terminology associated with TBI
  - medical aspects and recovery issues
  - severity classification systems
  - physical, cognitive, communicative, psychosocial outcomes frequently observed following TBI
  - prognostic factors

Similarities and differences between students with TBI and students with other types of handicapping conditions

- Target competencies
  - Educators will understand how this student is similar to or different from other student populations with which they are familiar
- Objective
  - to develop a frame of reference that will enable educators to compare and contrast what they currently know about

students with other handicapping conditions, such as learning disabilities, mental retardation, emotional disorders, behavioral disorders, physical impairments, and other health or learning disabilities with what they are learning about TBI
- Topics for discussion
  - diversity and variability within the TBI population
  - individual student's variability in performance and skill levels
  - premorbid educational history and performance

The impact of impairments resulting from TBI on the student's learning and performance

- Target competencies
  - Educators will associate performance and behaviors observed in the educational setting with impairments that have resulted from TBI
- Objectives
  - to identify student classroom performance and behaviors that are representative of impairments
  - to relate problems observed in the educational setting with impairments from the TBI
- Topics for discussion
  - learning problems and behaviors frequently observed in students with TBI
  - impact of impairments on learning capabilities, emotions, social interactions

–response patterns that may be representative of impairments resulting from TBI

Program decision making including policy and administration

- Target competencies
  - –Educators will understand the difficulties of fitting the student with TBI into the present scheme of educational programming given the current policies and guidelines under which schools must operate
- Objective
  - –to develop criteria for making educational programming decisions appropriate for meeting students' needs and in agreement with established local, state, and national guidelines and laws
- Topics for discussion
  - –educational programming during hospitalization
  - –networking between rehabilitation professionals and education professionals during hospitalization and rehabilitation, including roles and responsibilities of each discipline
  - –legal and ethical issues related to students' needs
  - –financial problems and constraints related to meeting students' needs
  - –classification and placement within the current educational framework and under the current educational guidelines

Educational program development including assessment and management strategies

- Target competencies
  - –Educators will understand how to develop effective programs based on the unique configuration of strengths and impairments presented by the student

with TBI, including assessment and management strategies
- Objectives
  - –to understand aspects of TBI that need to be considered during the assessment process
  - –to identify assessment techniques applicable to this population
  - –to incorporate assessment outcome data into the individualized education program
  - –to select appropriate teaching strategies, materials, and resources for instructing the student with TBI
- Topics for discussion
  - –skill areas to be assessed
  - –functional assessment strategies and methods
  - –support services frequently needed by students with TBI
  - –guidelines for making placement decisions
  - –specific instructional strategies and classroom adaptations appropriate for students' needs
  - –development of individualized education plans for students with TBI

Consultation and collaboration between professionals (rehabilitation and education) and with families for effective program planning

- Target competencies
  - –Educators will work cooperatively with other professionals (rehabilitation and education) to plan and implement programs
  - –Educators will meaningfully involve family and peers of students with TBI in program planning and implementation
- Objectives
  - –to implement a coordinated team approach to meet, to plan, and to implement programming for TBI students

–to share information and to exchange ideas with interdisciplinary team members and family about program planning and applicable assessment and management strategies

–to identify the most common family/peer issues and situations that interfere with school, vocational, and community reintegration

–to identify ethnic and cultural factors that may significantly impact program decision making

–to actively involve family in the IEP planning process by seeking their input regarding educational goals, placement, and teaching methodologies

- Topics for discussion

–consultation and collaboration as program approaches to meet the needs of this population

–the roles and responsibilities of various disciplines with regard to students with TBI (psychologists, speech-language pathologists, occupational therapists, physical therapists, educators, medical personnel, social workers, etc)

–the impact of TBI on the family

–the impact of TBI on relationships with peers

–strategies for incorporating family and peers into the planning process and program implementation

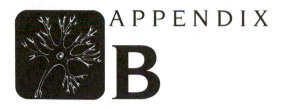

APPENDIX

B

Test Resources

Berg, E. A., & Grant, D. A. (1980). **The Wisconsin Card Sorting Test (WCST).** Odessa, FL: Psychological Assessment Resources, Inc.

Biery, K. E. (1982). **Developmental Test of Visual-Motor Integration.** Chicago, IL: Follett Publishing Company.

Buschke, H., & Fuld, P. A. (1974). Evaluating storage, retention, and retrieval in disordered memory and learning. **Neurology,** 1019–1025.

Carrow-Woolfolk, E. (1985). **Test for Auditory Comprehension of Language-Revised (TACL-R).** Allen, TX: DLM Teaching Resources.

Denckla, M. B., & Rudel, R. (1974). Rapid "automatized" naming (R.A.N.): Dyslexia differentiated from other learning disabilities. **Neuropsychologica, 14,** 471–479.

Denman, S. B. (1984). **Denman Neuropsychology Memory Scale.** Charleston, SC: Author.

DiSimoni, F. (1978). **The Token Test for Children.** Allen, TX: DLM Teaching Resources.

DiSimoni, F. (1989). **Comprehensive Apraxia Test.** Dalton, PA: Praxis House Publishers.

Dunn, L., & Dunn, L. (1981). **Peabody Picture Vocabulary Test-Revised (PPVT).** Minneapolis, MN: American Guidance Service.

Dunn, L., & Markwardt, F. C., Jr. (1970). **Peabody Individual Achievement Test (PIAT).** Circle Pines, MN: American Guidance Service.

Enderby, V., & Roworth, M. (1984). **Frenchay Dysarthria Assessment.** San Diego, CA: College-Hill Press.

Fisher's Auditory Problems Checklist. (1986). Bemidji, MN: LIFE Products.

Gardner, M. (1986). **Test of Visual-Motor Skills (TVMS) Ages 2 Years to 13 Years.** Burlingame, CA: Psychological and Educational Publications, Inc.

Gardner, M. (1992). **Test of Visual-Motor Skills: Upper Level Adolescents and Adults (TVMS:UL) Ages 12 Years to 40.** Burlingame, CA: Psychological and Educational Publications, Inc.

German, D. J. (1986). **Test of Word Finding.** Allen, TX: DLM Teaching Resources.

Hammill, D. (1985). **Detroit Tests of Learning Aptitude (DTLA-2).** Austin, TX: PRO-ED.

Hammill, D., & Larsen, S. C. (1988). **Test of Written Language-2 (TOWL-2).** Austin, TX: PRO-ED.

Hammill, D., & Newcomber, P. L. (1988). **Test of Language Development-2 Intermediate.** Austin, TX: PRO-ED.

Jorgenson, C., Barrett, M., Huisingh, R., & Zachman, L. (1981). **The Word Test.** Moline, IL: Lingui-Systems.

McCarney, S. B. (1986). **The Attention Deficit Disorders Evaluation Scale (ADDES).** Columbia, MO: Hawthorne Educational Services, Inc.

Newcomber, P. L., & Hammill, D. D. (1988). **Test of Language Development-2 (TOLD-2 Primary).** Austin, TX: PRO-ED.

Ross, D. (1986). **Ross Information Processing Assessment.** Austin, TX: PRO-ED.

Ross, J. D., & Ross, C. M. (1976). **Ross Test of Higher Cognitive Processes.** Novata, CA: Academic Therapy Publications.

Semel, E., Wiig, E. H., & Secord, W. (1987). **Clinical Evaluation of Language Fundamentals-Revised (CELF-R).** San Antonio, TX: The Psychological Corporation.

Shearer, B. (1992). **Hillside Assessment of Pre-Trauma Intelligence (HAPI).** Warren, OH: Hillside Rehabilitation Hospital.

Woodcock, R., & Johnson, M. (1989). **Woodcock-Johnson Psycho-Educational Test Battery.** Allen Park, TX: DLM Teaching Resources.

Zachman, L., Barrett, M., Huisingh, R., Orman, S., & Blagden, C. (1991). **The Adolescent Test of Problem Solving (TOPS).** East Moline, IL: Lingui-Systems.

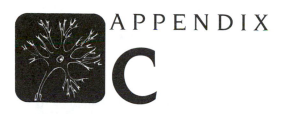

APPENDIX C

References for Resource Materials

Adaptive Communication
  Systems, Inc.
354 Hookstown Grade Road
Clinton, Pennsylvania 15206

Attention Process Training
  (ATP)
Association for Neuropsycho-
  logical Research and
  Development
Puyallup, Washington 98371

Brain Train
Rehabilitation Psychology
  Associates
P.O. Box 1510
Beaverton, Oregon 97075-1510

Cannon Corporation
One Cannon Plaza
Lake Success, New York 11042

Communication Skill Builders
3630 E. Bellevue
P.O. Box 42050-E92
Tuscon, Arizona 85733

DLM
1 DLM Park
Allen, Texas 75002

Disney Comic Strip Maker
Disney Educational Software
Sunburst Communications
P.O. Box 2000
Thornwood, New Jersey 10594

Imaginart Communication
  Products
307 Arizona Street
Bisbee, Arizona 85603

Lingui-Systems
3100 Fourth Avenue
E. Moline, Illinois 61244

Midwest Publications
P.O. Bo 448
Pacific Grove, California 93950

Milton Bradley
Springfield, Massachusetts 01101

Mayer-Johnson Company
P.O. Box AD
Solana Beach, California 92075-
0838

Prentke-Romich
1022 Heyl Road
Wooster, Ohio 44691

PRO-ED
8700 Shoal Boulevard
Austin, Texas 78758-6897

Self-Esteem in the Classroom
Jack Canfield
Self Esteem Seminars
17156 Palisades Circle
Pacific Palisades, California
90272

Sentient Systems Technology
5001 Baum Boulevard
Pittsburgh, Pennsylvania 15123

Speech Bin
8 Beechtree Lane
Plainboro, New Jersey 08536

Stickey Bear
Weekley Reader Family Software
Middletown, Connecticut 06457
Towards Affective Development
(TAD)
American Guidance Service
Circle Plains, Minnesota 55014

Thinking Publications
7021 West Lower Creek Road
Eau Claire, Wisconsin 54701

Visiting Nurse Service
1200 McArthur Drive
Akron, Ohio 44320

Words+, Inc.
P.O. Box 1229
Lancaster, California 93535

Zygo Industries, Inc.
P.O. Box 1008
Portland, Oregon 97207

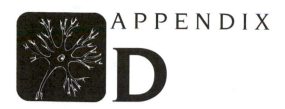

D

Cognitive-Communication Areas: General Behaviors, Social Behaviors, Expressive Language, Receptive Language, and Written Language

General Behaviors

Impairment	Classroom Behaviors	Skills and Teaching Strategies
Decreased judgment.	Easily persuaded by others (can be convinced by others to act inappropriately; abuses drugs and alcohol).	*Decision Making*: Select a classroom buddy to keep the students aware of instructions, class rules, appropriate social conduct.
	Impulsive	Establish a system of verbal or nonverbal signals to cue the student to alter behavior (call the student's name, touch him or her, use a written sign or hand signal).
	Speaks out-of-turn in class, gets up and moves about the classroom.	*Self-Monitoring*: Establish specific rules for behavior in certain places and times of the day; practice implementation frequently in controlled situations before allowing the child to do something independently.
	Careless about safety. Does not look before crossing streets; poor decisions about playing on the playground equipment or in activities in physical education class.	*Self-Awareness*: Make the student aware of the need for supervision (e.g. motoric problem, safety, etc.).
	Unreasonable demands to be unsupervised (wants to begin driving, again, too soon).	Establish small steps for progress toward greater independence.

Impairment	Classroom Behaviors	Skills and Teaching Strategies
Lacks self-insight.	Doesn't understand the rationale behind another person's reactions to behavior; paranoid.	*Awareness Of Self And Others*: Explain the cause for the other person's reaction.
		Explain what would have been a better way to behave (need simplistic explanations; reasoning will not help).
	Responds defensively to comments made or questions asked by teachers and other students.	Do not react or respond as if you need to prove a point; avoid confrontation; avoid "buying into" the argument.
Poor problem-solving skills.	Solutions to situations are not carefully thought through.	*Problem Solving*: Ask questions designed to help the student identify the problem, plan out and organize implementation or a solution.
Unable to plan for the future.	No recognition that there is a physical or cognitive problem or that there should be limitations to taking classes or performing tasks.	*Self-Awareness*: Plan activities that are similar in nature to what other classmates are doing, but adjust the level of complexity to the student's limitations.
		Build on success rather than make the student feel like a failure.

General *Behaviors (continued)*

Impairment	Classroom Behaviors	Skills and Teaching Strategies
Recognition.	No recognition of due dates or amount of time it would take to complete a class project.	*Organization & Planning:* Help the student formulate and use a system for maintaining organization. Require the student to carry a written log of activities, schedule of classes, list of assignments and due dates, and map of room locations. Frequently monitor the student's use of the organization system.
	Forget to prepare for a field trip.	
	Cannot predetermine materials needed for completing class projects (material, thread, pattern for home economics)	
Decreased carryover for new learning.	Information presented in class on Day 1 will not be recalled or generalized on Day 3.	*Compensatory Memory Strategies:* Teach the student to categorize, associate, rehearse, chunk information. Require the student to write things. Assign a student buddy to monitor and check what has been written.
Decreased ability to generalize learned information to new or different situations.	Unable to take tests for which newly learned information must be applied or generalized.	*Memory & Recall Strategies:* Recognize that this skill is not likely to improve, as change may not occur. Provide the student with a variety of examples of the topic or information to be tested.
Decreased ability to store and retrieve information upon demand.	Little or no attention to details in deductive reasoning tasks.	*Identifying Details:* Use visual and auditory cues to draw attention to details (highlight, underline, use reference pictures).
	Unable to recall specific details of a history lesson or all of the critical elements of a science experiment.	

Impairment	Classroom Behaviors	Skills and Teaching Strategies
Decreased judgment		
Lacks self insight		
Poor problem solving skills		
Unable to plan for the future		
Decreased carryover for new learning		
Increased ability to generalize learned information to new or different situations		
Increased ability to store and retrieve information upom demand		

Note: This form is for the reader's use.

Social Behaviors

Impairment	Classroom Behaviors	Skills and Teaching Strategies
Inability to perform well in competitive and stressful situations.	Argues and fights with peers on the playground.	*Sharing:* Select a classroom buddy with whom the child already gets along. Introduce sharing during small group activities; gradually include in full classroom activities; repeat the same procedure from individual to small group to large group on the playground.
Subtle noncompliance of classroom rules and activities.	Withdrawn and not willing to participate in group activities, such as work on a science project, small group discussion. Refuses to recite in class even when called on.	*Initiating Self-Concept:* Begin to elicit responses from the student during individual and seat work activities when you can be assured that the student can be correct; gradually request occasional responses in front of the student's friends, then small groups; repeat until the student feels comfortable participating in a large group.
Rude, silly, immature.	Makes nasty and/or inappropriate comments to fellow students and teachers.	*Judgment:* Present the student with "what if . . ." situations and choices.
	Laughs out loud during serious discussions or quiet seat work.	Give the student opportunities to verbally express judgment and decision making regarding appropriate behavior as well as opportunities role play.

Impairment	Classroom Behaviors	Skills and Teaching Strategies
Aggressive (verbal).	Interrupts conversations between fellow classmates.	*Turntaking:* Teach the student to concentrate on the comments of others.
		Nonverbally cue the student to discontinue interruptive behaviors.
Lacks initiative.	Homework is forgotten, not completed, or not turned in.	*Memory Task Completion Responsibility:* Develop, with the student, a daily written assignment sheet indicating dates and times assignments are due.
Unable to stay on task.	Unable to begin and/or complete timed math tests.	*Attention/Concentration:* Remove distractions: verbally cue the student to "begin" a task; nonverbally regain the student's attention and direct it to the required task.
	Unable to sit still in class while others are busy doing seat work or taking notes.	
	Goes from one assignment to the next, unable to complete either one, skips around while doing an assignment, completing only parts of it.	

Social Behaviors (continued)

Impairment	Classroom Behaviors	Skills and Teaching Strategies
Low frustration tolerance.	Displays an outburst of temper when others would try a different approach or request help	*Self-Awareness Of Internal Stress*: Do not attempt to punish the behavior using traditional behavior management approaches
		Learn to detect behaviors leading up to an outburst and intervene prior to it happening (watch the student's body language).
		Allow time for the student to be away from the situation and get needed rest or emotional release.
		Provide an understanding person with whom the student can share feelings and frustrations.
Inconsistent performance.	Homework on Day 1 is 100% correct, on Day 2 it is incorrect.	*Self-Monitoring*: Inform the student of errors made and why they were made.
	Demonstrates model behavior one day and totally inappropriate behavior the next.	When giving an assignment, let the student know the similarities to previous work that has been completed successfully.

Impairment	Classroom Behaviors	Skills and Teaching Strategies
Inability to perform well in competitive or stressful situations		
Subtle non-compliance of classroom rules and activities		
Rude, silly, immature		
Agressive (verbal)		
Lacks initiative		
Unable to stay on task		
Inconsistent performance		

Note: This form is for the reader's use.

Expressive Language

Impairment	Classroom Behaviors	Skills and Teaching Strategies
Demonstrates a difference between communication in informal situations and formal situations, such as the classroom.	Answers teacher's questions at a surface level; when pressed to give reasons why or more detail, student is unable to provide more info.	*Providing Adequate & Substantial Info.:* Direct the amount and type of information provided by the student. Encourage conversations to develop by giving instructions such as "Tell me more"; "How many did you see..." Role Play formal conversations in small groups.
Length of sentences and use of gestures may be normal; depth of communication is not.	Although appearing to do quite well conversationally during social situations, classroom speaking lacks detail and depth.	Direct the context of the student's responses with your own verbal models, cues, and leading questions. *Storage & Retrieval Of Information:* Teach memory strategies (rehearsal, chunking, visualization, association, etc...).
Communication is tangential (rambling).	Conversations tend to ramble with no acknowledgment of the listener's interest or attention.	*Topic Maintenance:* When the student begins to deviate from the topic, either provide a nonverbal cue or stop the youngster so he or she doesn't continue in front of classmates. Teach the student to recognize nonverbal behaviors indicating lack of interest or desire to make a comment. (Work with this skill during private conversations with the student.)
	Conversation may be topic-related but not exactly what is desired or key to the discussion (ex: when asked to name the major food groups, the student might begin a discussion about irrigation and growing crops).	Teach beginning, middle, end of stories. Stop the student's response and restate the original question; focusing the student's attention on the key issues.

Impairment	Classroom Behaviors	Skills and Teaching Strategies
Word retrieval errors.	Answers contain a high use of "this," "that," "those things," "whatchamacallits."	*Word Recall*: Teach the student association skills and to give definitions of words he or she cannot recall.
	Difficulty providing answers on fill-in-the-blank tests.	Teach memory strategies (rehearsal, association, visualization, etc.).
Verbal problem-solving ability is reduced.	In algebra class, the student may arrive at a correct answer but not be able to recite the steps followed to solve the problem.	*Problem-Solving*: Teach inductive and deductive reasoning at appropriate age levels.
Poor reasoning skills.		*Reasoning*: Privately (not during classroom situations or in front or peers) ask the student to explain answers and provide reasons.
Reduced ability to use abstractness in conversation (ambiguity, satire, inferences, drawing conclusions).	Says things that classmates interpret as satirical, funny, or bizarre, although not intended to be that way.	*Semantics*: Teach the student common phrases used for satire, idioms, puns and so on.
Delayed responses	When called on to give an answer, the student will not answer immediately, appearing not to know the answer.	*Processing*: Allow extra time for the student to discuss and explain.
		Avoid asking too many questions.

Expressive Language *(continued)*

Impairment	Classroom Behaviors	Skills and Teaching Strategies
Unable to describe events in appropriate detail and sequence.	When relating an experience, details are out of order, confused, or overlapping.	*Sequencing:* Teach sequencing skills.
	Can't explain to another student the directions for playing a game in physical education class.	Direct the context of the student's responses.
Inadequate labeling or vocabulary to convey clear messages.	Inappropriately labels tools in industrial arts class.	*Semantics:* Teach the student vocabulary associated with specific subject areas and classroom activities.

Impairment	Classroom Behaviors	Skills and Teaching Strategies
Demonstrates a difference between communication in informal situations and formal situations such as the classroom.		
Length of sentences and use of gestures may be normal; depth of communication is not.		
Communication is tangential (rambling)		
Word retrieval errors.		
Verbal problem solving ability is reduced.		
Poor reasoning skills		
Reduced ability to use abstractions in conversation (ambiguity, satire, inferences, drawing conclusions) Delayed responses.		
Unable to describe events in appropriate detail and sequence.		
Inadequate labeling or vocabulary to convey clear messages.		

Note: This form is for the reader's use.

Receptive Language

Impairment	Classroom Behaviors	Skills and Teaching Strategies
Unable to determine salient features.	Completes the wrong assignment. (Teacher requested that the class complete problems 9–12, this student completes problems 1–12.)	*Organization*: Encourage the student to write assignments in his daily log.
Unable to determine specific aspects of questions.	When answering questions about the details of a history lesson, gets the details confused.	*Finding the Facts*: Ask questions which will elicit the student's recall of important facts.
	When asked specific question, responses may be related but not exact.	
	Unable to decipher long story problems.	
Unable to mentally organize information presented verbally or in written form.	Performs steps of the science project out of sequence either fixating on 1 step or performing the most apparent step. ("I know the other steps, I just didn't need to do them.")	*Sequencing*: Provide the student with written 3 & 4 step sequences to sort and organize. Do not allow the student to skip steps in a demonstration even if he says he or she knows what to do.
Unable to analyze and integrate information received.	Executes written directions in an unorganized and incomplete manner.	*Direction Following*: Directions should be written in 1, 2, 3, and so on . . . steps rather than in paragraph form.
	Goes to the gymnasium for a program when it was announced that it would be held in the auditorium.	

Impairment	Classroom Behaviors	Skills and Teaching Strategies
Easily over-loaded by high amounts of oral information presented during classroom instruction.	Appears to be daydreaming and nonresponsive while the teacher is lecturing or giving instruction.	*Focus Attention*: Use pauses when giving classroom instructions to allow for processing information. Use short, simple sentences when explaining information.
Unable to read non-verbal cues of others.	Unaware that the teacher or other classmates do not want to be bothered while they are working.	*Social Awareness*: Use preestablished non-verbal cues to alert the student that his or her behavior is inappropriate. Explain what was wrong with the behavior and what would have been appropriate.
Difficulty comprehending spoken messages if presented in terms, rapidly, or lengthy.	Exhibits poor notetaking skills, unable to maintain the ability to sort out and note the important parts of the teacher's discussion.	*Comprehension*: Use short, simple sentences emphasizing key points by voice variations, intonations and so on. Alert the student to the important topic being discussed.

Receptive Language (continued)

Impairment	Classroom Behaviors	Skills and Teaching Strategies
Difficulty understanding or recognizing a sequence of events.	Even after being back to school for a while, still gets lost in the daily routine of the school day (knowing that spelling follows math, etc...)	*Organization:* Provide the student with a written schedule of the youngster's school routine and map of the rooms he or she must get to.
Difficulty maintaining attention and concentration.	Loses place while reading; unable to relate information recently read; easily distracted during reading assignments; unable to complete silent reading and seatwork assignments at the same rate as classmates.	*Processing:* Provide with additional time to complete classroom and homework tasks.
		Attention Concentration: Because the student will most likely be processing at the best rate he or she can, provide with ample time for reading assignments.
		Reduce the amount of work to be read by assigning summaries, and so on.
Unable to understand abstractness in others' language (satire, puns).	Misunderstands instructions and comments make while classmates are responding to satire, jokes, puns, and so on. The student appears to be unaware of what is so funny.	*Semantics:* Do not use satire and such when presenting important information, teaching, or trying to correct the student's behavior.
		Teach the student the meaning of idioms, figurative language, ambiguous phrases, and so on.

Impairment	Classroom Behaviors	Skills and Teaching Strategies
Unable to determine salient features.		
Unable to determine specific aspects of questions.		
Word retrieval errors.		
Unable to mentally organize information presented verbally or in written form.		
Unable to analyze and integrate information received.		
Unable to read non-verbal cues of others.		
Difficulty comprehending spoken messages if presented in terms, rapidly, or lengthy.		
Difficulty maintaining attention and concentration.		
Unable to understand abstractness in others' language (satire, puns).		

Note: This form is for the reader's use.

Written Language

Impairment	Classroom Behaviors	Skills and Teaching Strategies
Structure and content of writing may not be at the same level as preinjury.	Answers to essay test may contain numerous grammatical errors, sentence structure is incorrect and unorganized.	*Syntactic Complexity:* Give the student time to go over written work with a partner or teaching aide to find and correct errors.
Demonstrates simplistic sentence structure and syntactic disorganization.	Sentences used and topics discussed are simplistic when compared to expectations for age and grade. Themes may be short and dry.	*Proofreading & Semantics:* Provide the student with the worksheets which focus on teaching vocabulary, grammar, and proofreading skills.
Content of writing is very literal, devoid of figurative language; contains irrelevancies and unsubstantiated information.	Description of a science project contains several nonessential details.	*Providing Adequate & Substantial Information & Sequencing & Expressing Ideas Through Writing:* Allow the student to verbally state ideas, taperecord, and write from dictation.
	If asked to write a theme about a major issue in government class, the paper will contain several issue assertions with no evidence to support the assertion.	Present the student with "question cards", indicating the specific issues that are to be addressed in an essay or discussed in a theme.
	Essays written following the injury lack the same flair, creativity noted prior to the injury.	Accept that there will be a difference in skill level pre- and postinjury. Work at the student's level and ability.
Speed and accuracy are decreased; poor legibility.	Performance on timed tests in math is slower than that of other classmates.	*Check Work For Accuracy:* Accept that the student will take longer to complete assignments; reduce and alter the requirements.
Poor planning of use of space on the paper.	Care is not given to the appearance of work.	*Spatial Relationships:* Utilize art teaching methodology to help the student identify and correct problems.
	When making posters or art projects, sizes of pictures are disproportionate or located inappropriately on the paper.	Understand that physical capabilities may be limiting writing skills. Reteach, if appropriate for age and grade.

Impairment	Classroom Behaviors	Skills and Teaching Strategies
Structure and content of writing may not be at the same level as preinjury		
Demonstrates simplistic sentence structure and syntactic disorganization		
Content of writing is very literal, devoid of figurative language; contains irrelevancies and unsubstantiated information		
Poor planning of use of space on paper		

Note: This form is for the reader's use.

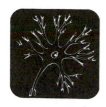

Index